Gone Grazy®

Everyday Grazing Boards

JANICE GERGES

Written by: Dietitian Zain ul Abedin

Designed by: Anila Adnan

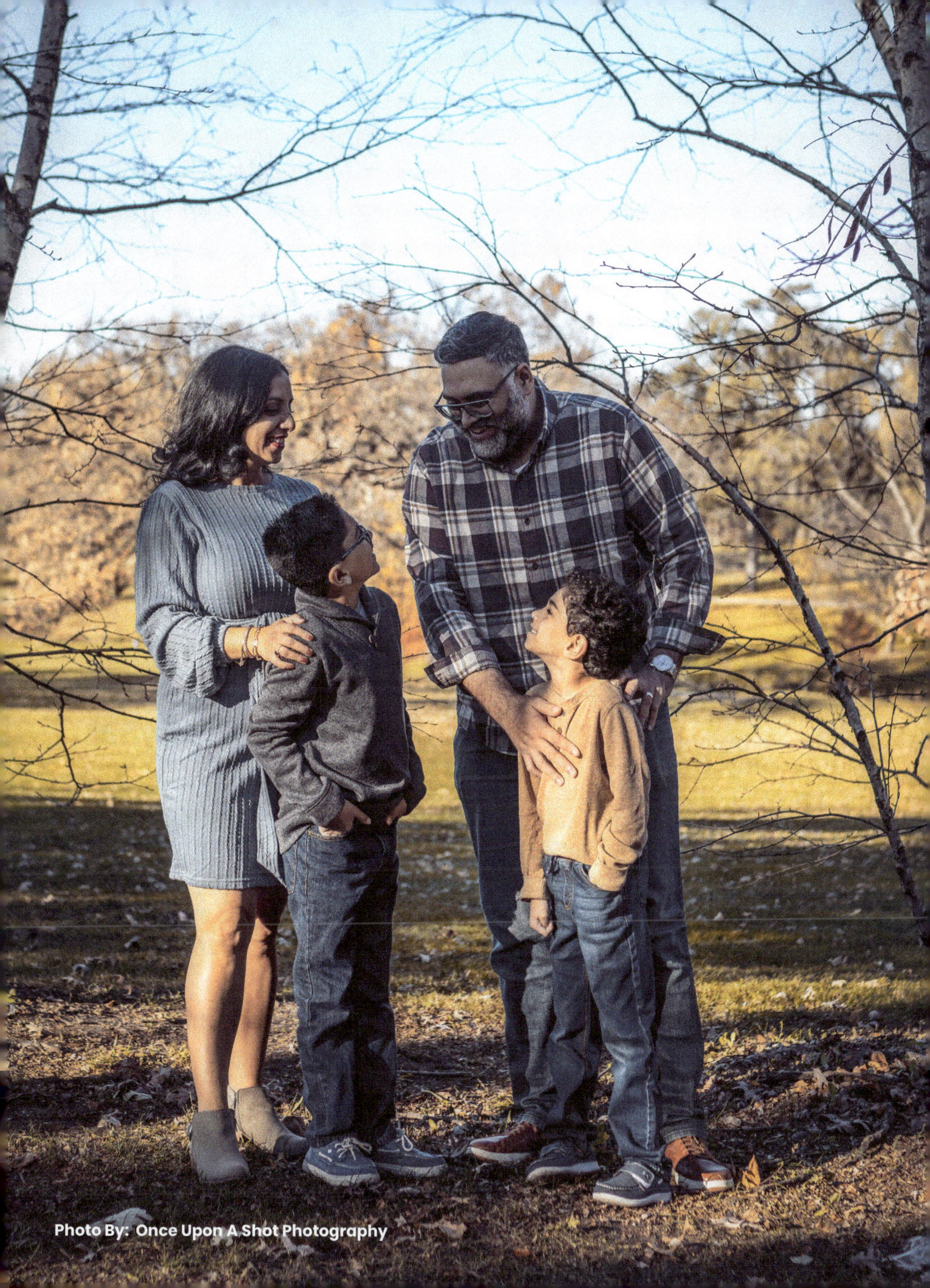

Table of Contents

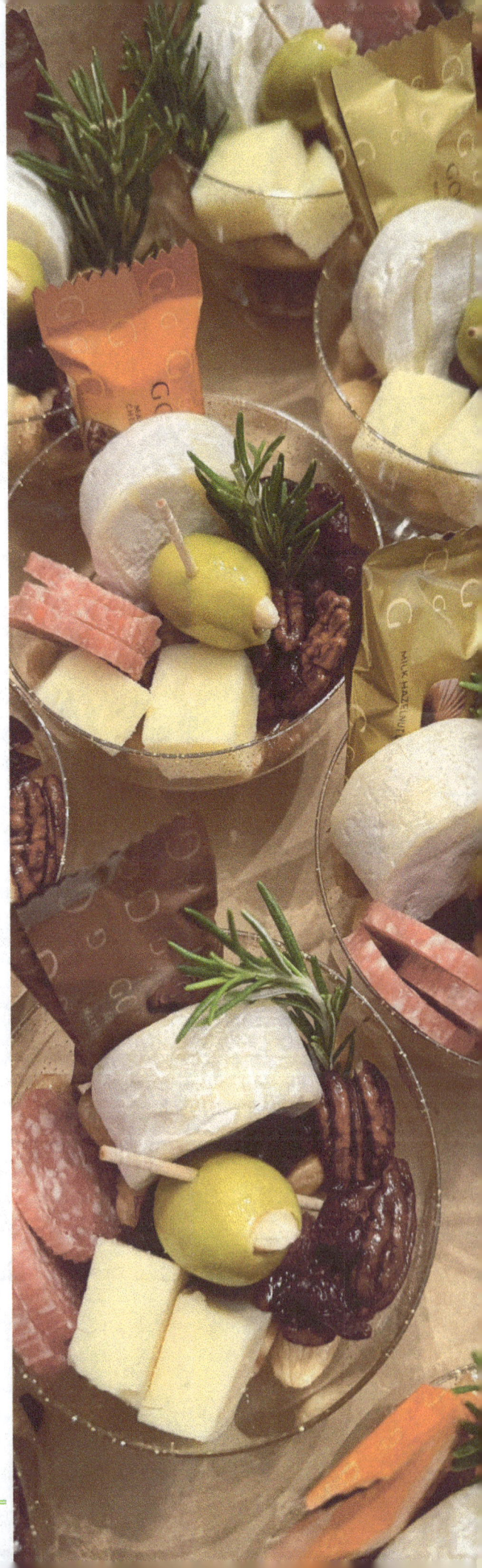

The board that started it all...

Football has always been one of my favorite sports to watch. Combined with my love of food and hosting family & friends, this was a board I made at home in February of 2021 while watching Super Bowl LV, amidst the global pandemic.

Details and themes are my favorites! I love a fun occasion, party or really any excuse to share food with loved ones. I have realized the details come naturally to me, like slicing pretzel buns into quarters to create a football shape and using shelled pistachios to resemble a grassy football field. I'm often asked if I plan my boards in advance, and I do not! I'm just sure to have plenty of food and snacks on hand, and then I run with it. We didn't have a big party that day as we normally would, but naturally, I shared this photo with friends and received many compliments. That same weekend, a friend encouraged me to make her a board and officially launch my local grazing business, Gone Grazy®. I simultaneously started an Instagram page and was delighted to find that my wonderful friends and neighbors began telling people they knew about my boards (they haven't stopped)!

After receiving numerous positive responses to this board and many others, and listening to people tell me I have a talent and that I'm creative, I started believing that I was on to something with food art. I don't take compliments well – I get that awkward feeling of not knowing what to do with them or how to respond. But the overwhelming support and encouragement certainly have motivated me so much that I'm opening my first brick-and-mortar storefront location in 2024!

My hope for you reading this book is to also feel confident and inspired by these ideas to put your own creative spin on food...board it and they will come!

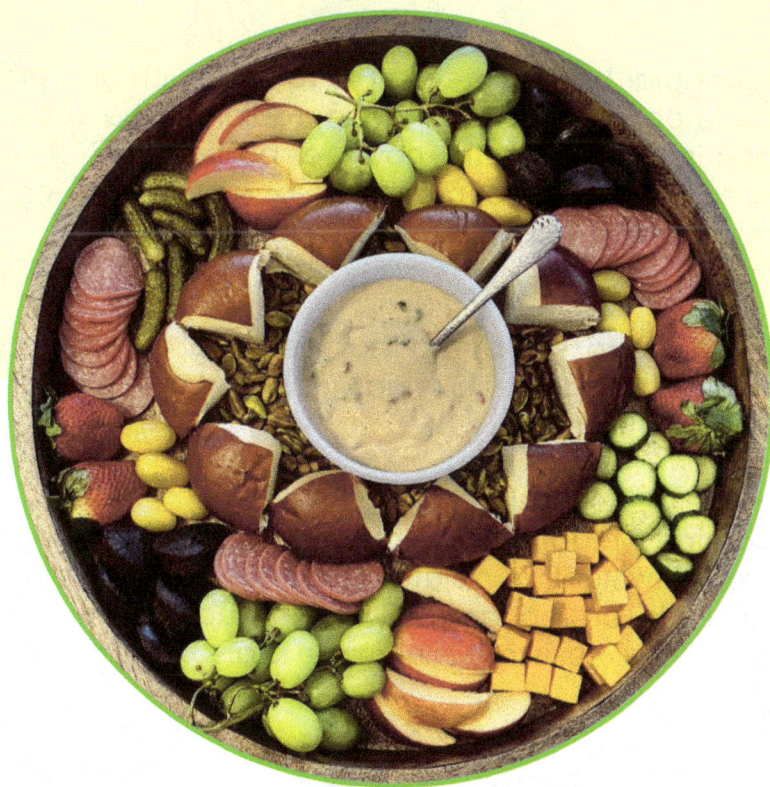

Introduction

Creating a beautiful and functional charcuterie or snack board begins with selecting the right base. The type of board you choose can significantly impact the presentation and overall experience.

Choose Your Board

There are so many shapes and styles of charcuterie boards that it can be a little overwhelming. Check out our tips for choosing the right board:

Shape

Rectangular boards are simple to work with and provide an excellent surface on which to arrange ingredients. The second most common shape is a round board, however portion control with these is a little trickier. Once you've mastered a rectangular or round board, try experimenting with different shapes.

Size

For a standard-size board that feeds 4 to 6 guests, go with something around 8" x 12" or 9" x 13". A larger board with a length over 18" or 20" is suitable for a crowd.

Material

Melamine breadboards are a convenient option because they are more lightweight than slate or wood boards, but they provide the same rustic look. Large boards with many ingredients tend to become very heavy. Break-resistant melamine is also safe for your patio or outdoor dining space.

Types of Boards

Here's an overview of the various types of boards available and the benefits of each:

1. Wooden Boards

Wooden boards are a classic choice for charcuterie and snack displays. Made from materials such as bamboo, acacia, or walnut, these boards offer a warm, rustic appeal that complements a variety of food items. Wooden boards are durable and come in numerous shapes and sizes, making them versatile for any occasion. They are perfect for presenting cheeses, meats, fruits, and more.

Where to Buy: Williams Sonoma, Crate & Barrel, Amazon, Etsy

Care Instructions: Hand wash with warm, soapy water. Avoid soaking and never put in the dishwasher. Periodically oil with food-safe mineral oil to prevent drying and cracking.

2. Marble Boards

Marble boards exude elegance and sophistication, making them ideal for upscale gatherings. Because marble naturally retains heat, they are especially helpful for keeping cheeses and other perishables cold. Marble boards are available in various colors and patterns, adding a touch of luxury to your presentation.

Where to Buy: West Elm, Bed Bath & Beyond, Wayfair, Amazon

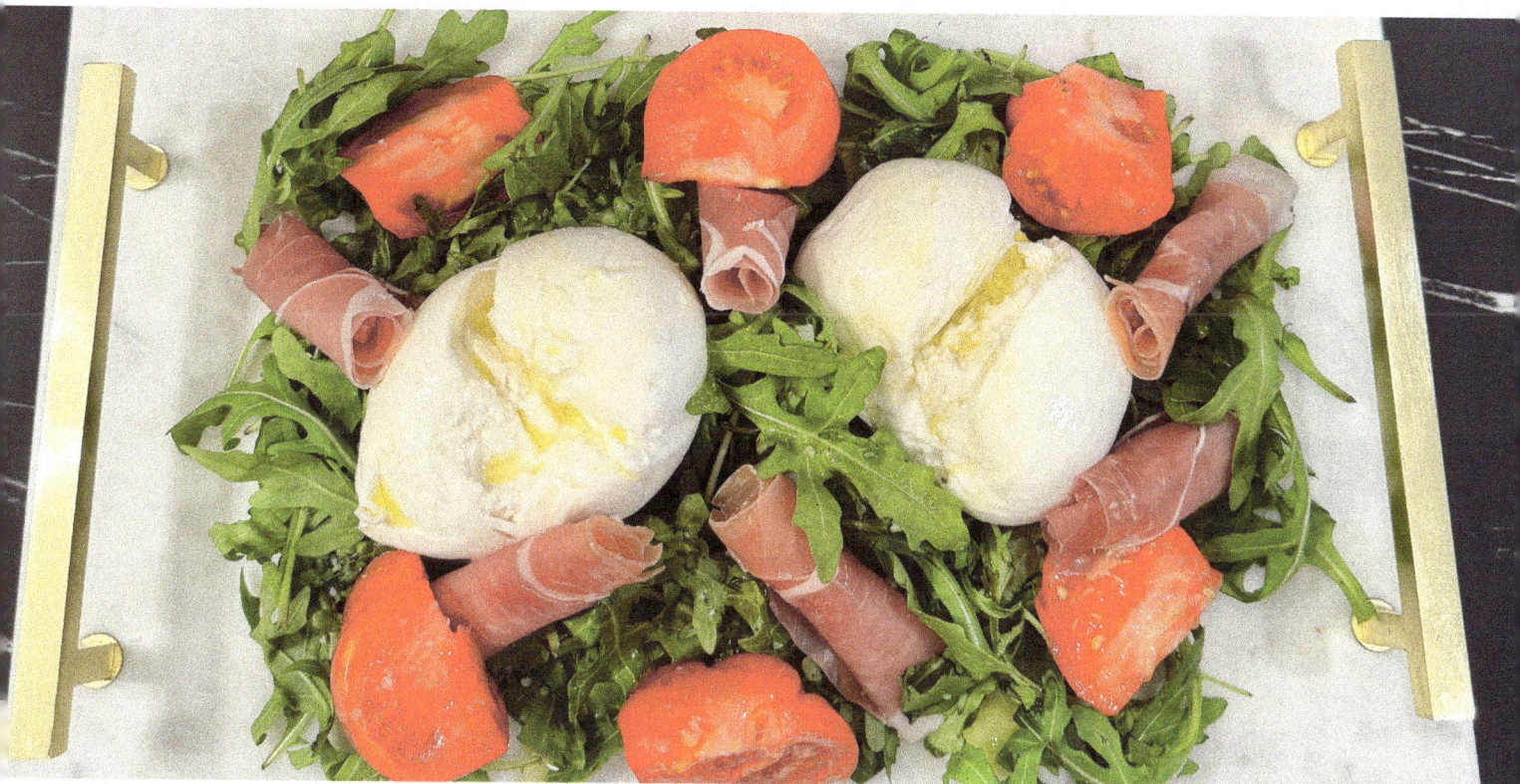

Care Instructions: Wipe with a damp cloth and mild detergent. Avoid abrasive cleaners. Do not submerge in water or put in the dishwasher.

3. Slate Boards
Slate boards offer a sleek and modern look, perfect for contemporary presentations. One unique feature of slate is its writable surface, which allows you to label different items with chalk—a fun and practical touch for guests. These boards are excellent for serving cheeses, charcuterie, and appetizers.

Where to Buy: Target, West Elm, Amazon, Uncommon Goods

Care Instructions: Hand wash with warm water and mild soap. Do not put in the dishwasher. Allow to air dry completely before storing.

4. Plastic Boards
Plastic or melamine boards are lightweight, durable, and available in a variety of colors and designs. Their durability and ease of cleaning make them ideal for outdoor gatherings, picnics, and kid-friendly snack boards. These boards are quite practical and reasonably priced.
Where to Buy: Walmart, IKEA, Amazon

Care Instructions: Most plastic boards are dishwasher safe, but hand washing can extend their life. Avoid using abrasive scrubbers.

5. Glass Boards
Glass boards are non-porous and easy to clean, making them a hygienic choice for food presentation. They give your setup a slick touch and come in clear and attractive styles. Glass boards are perfect for showcasing cheeses, fruits, and desserts.

Where to Buy: Macy's, Bed Bath & Beyond, Amazon

Care Instructions: Dishwasher safe, but hand washing is recommended to prevent chipping. Use a soft cloth to avoid scratches.

6. Ceramic Boards
Ceramic boards are stylish and often used for presenting cheeses and desserts. Available in various colors and patterns, these boards add an artistic flair to your display. They are sturdy and provide a solid base for an array of food items.

Where to Buy: Pottery Barn, Wayfair, Amazon

Care Instructions: Hand wash with warm, soapy water. Avoid harsh abrasives and extreme temperature changes to prevent cracking.

Board Care and Maintenance

General Cleaning Tips

» After each use, scrape off any leftover food and rinse the board with warm water.
» Use a mild dish soap and a soft sponge or cloth to clean the surface.
» Immediately dry with a fresh towel after rinsing well to avoid warping and moisture absorption.

Deep Cleaning

» Periodically massage with a half-lemon and sprinkle coarse salt over the surface of wooden and bamboo boards. This aids in odor removal and disinfection.
» For marble and slate boards, create a paste of baking soda and water for a gentle scrub. Rinse well and dry completely.
» For plastic and glass boards, a mixture of vinegar and water can be used for deeper cleaning and sanitizing.

Avoiding Damage

» Do not soak wooden, marble, or slate boards in water, as prolonged exposure can cause damage.
» Avoid using harsh or abrasive cleaners on any board material to prevent surface damage.
» Keep boards away from extreme temperatures and direct sunlight, which can cause warping or cracking.

Storage Tips

» Store boards upright in a cool, dry place to prevent warping.
» Every few months, lightly treat wooden boards with mineral oil that is appropriate for food use to maintain moisture and prevent drying out.
» Keep boards away from direct heat sources, such as stoves or ovens, to prolong their lifespan.

Dip Bowls and Serving Utensils

Your charcuterie and snack board presentation can be enhanced by not only selecting the ideal board but also by employing the appropriate small dip bowls and serving utensils, which offer both flair and functionality. This is a list of some necessary items:

Small Dip Bowls (Ramekins)

Small dip bowls, or ramekins, are perfect for containing sauces, dips, spreads, and smaller items that might otherwise roll around on your board. They keep everything neat and prevent mixing of flavors.

» **Materials:** Common materials for ramekins include ceramic, porcelain, glass, and stainless steel. Ceramic and porcelain ramekins offer a classic look, while glass and stainless steel add a modern touch.
» **Sizes:** Available in various sizes, typically ranging from 2 to 6 oz. Choose the size based on the type and quantity of dip you're serving.

Honey Dippers

Honey dippers are an essential tool for drizzling honey over cheeses, fruits, or nuts. Their unique design helps control the flow of honey, allowing you to add just the right amount without making a mess.

» **Materials**: Stainless steel and wood are typical choices. While stainless steel is sleek and contemporary, wooden dippers have a rustic feel to them.

Cheese Knives

Cheese knives come in various shapes and sizes, each designed to handle different types of cheese. Having a selection of these knives on your board makes it easier for guests to serve themselves while keeping the presentation clean.

Types:

» **Soft Cheese Knife:** Features a thin blade with holes, reducing the surface area to prevent soft cheeses from sticking.
» **Hard Cheese Knife:** Sturdy and pointed for cutting through firm cheeses like cheddar or gouda.
» **Spreaders:** Used for creamy cheeses and spreads like Brie or goat cheese.

Cheese Spreaders

Cheese spreaders are ideal for serving soft cheeses, pâtés, or spreads. Their broad, flat blade is designed to scoop and spread smoothly without tearing bread or crackers.

» **Materials:** Available in stainless steel, wood, and sometimes paired with ceramic or resin handles for decorative flair.

Tongs

When picking up little items like olives, pickles, or small fruits, tongs come in handy. They offer a hygienic way for guests to serve themselves without touching the food directly.

» **Materials:** Stainless steel, silicone, and bamboo are common. Silicone-tipped tongs are gentle on delicate items, while stainless steel provides durability.

Serving Spoons and Forks

Miniature serving spoons and forks are great for dips, spreads, and small appetizers. They add an extra layer of elegance to your board while providing practicality.

» **Materials:** Stainless steel, wood, and bamboo. Stainless steel is durable and easy to clean, while wood and bamboo offer a more rustic, natural look.

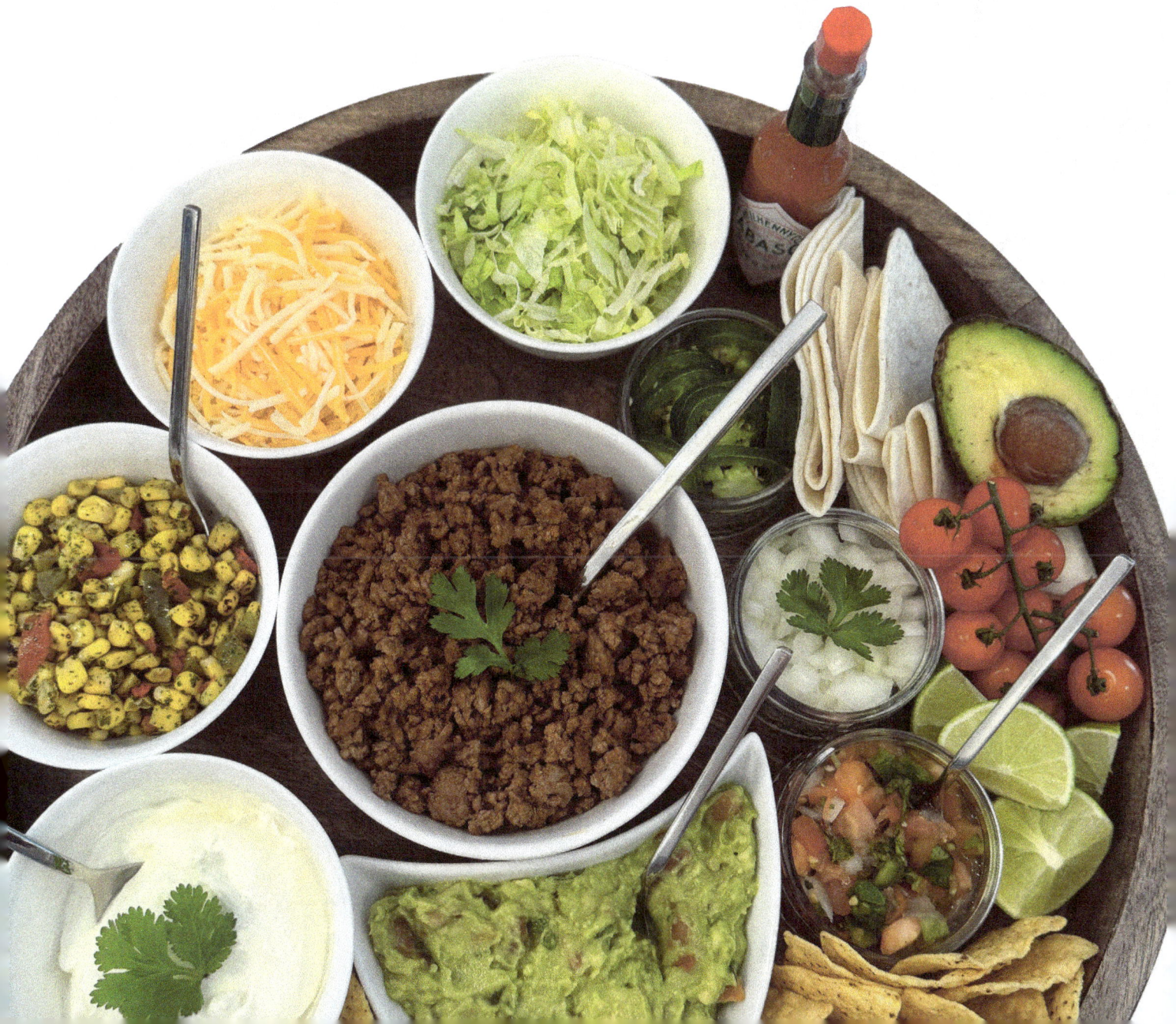

Kids Snack Board

🦋 Preparation time
5 minutes

🔔 Serving
6-7 kids

Ingredients:

» 7 sausage sticks
» 1 cup pepperoni slices
» 1 cup Colby cheese cubes
» 20 RITZ crackers
» 1 cucumber
» 8 baby carrots
» 8 Babybel cheese cube pieces.
» 6 chocolate chip cookies
» 1 cup Goldfish crackers
» 1 cup peanut butter filled pretzels
» 1 sliced apple.

Instructions:

1. Wash and slice the cucumbers and apples.
2. On a large platter or board, arrange the sausage sticks, pepperoni slices, and Colby cheese cubes.
3. Align RITZ crackers along the board.
4. Place the Goldfish crackers, and peanut butter-filled pretzels in small bowls on the board.
5. Add the sliced cucumbers, baby carrots, and Babybel cheese cubes around the board.
6. Position the chocolate chip cookies and sliced apples in separate sections.
7. Organize everything so that it is easily accessible.
8. Serve immediately or cover and refrigerate until ready to serve.

Tips
Arrange the ingredients in a colorful pattern to make the board visually appealing for kids. Use small cookie cutters to create fun shapes from the cheese or cucumber slices.

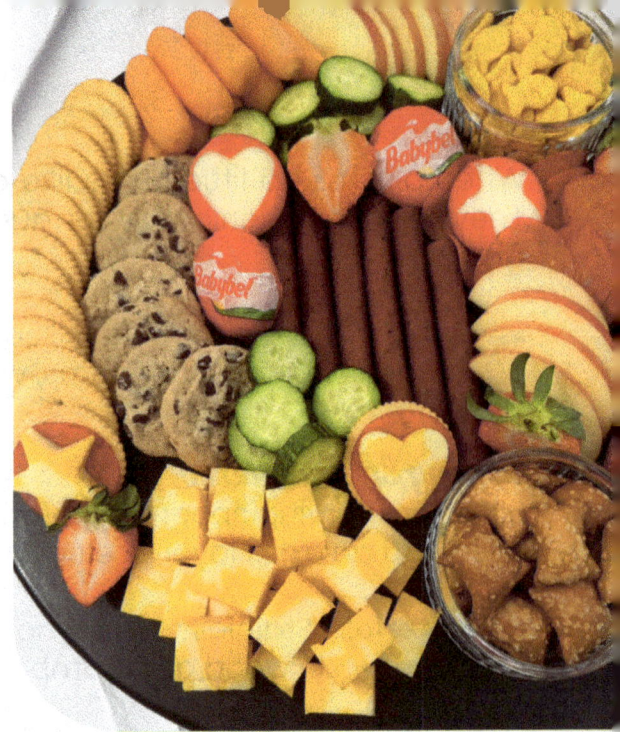

Nutrition facts (per serving)

Calories: 425cal,	Carbs: 30g,	Protein: 12g,	Fat: 25g

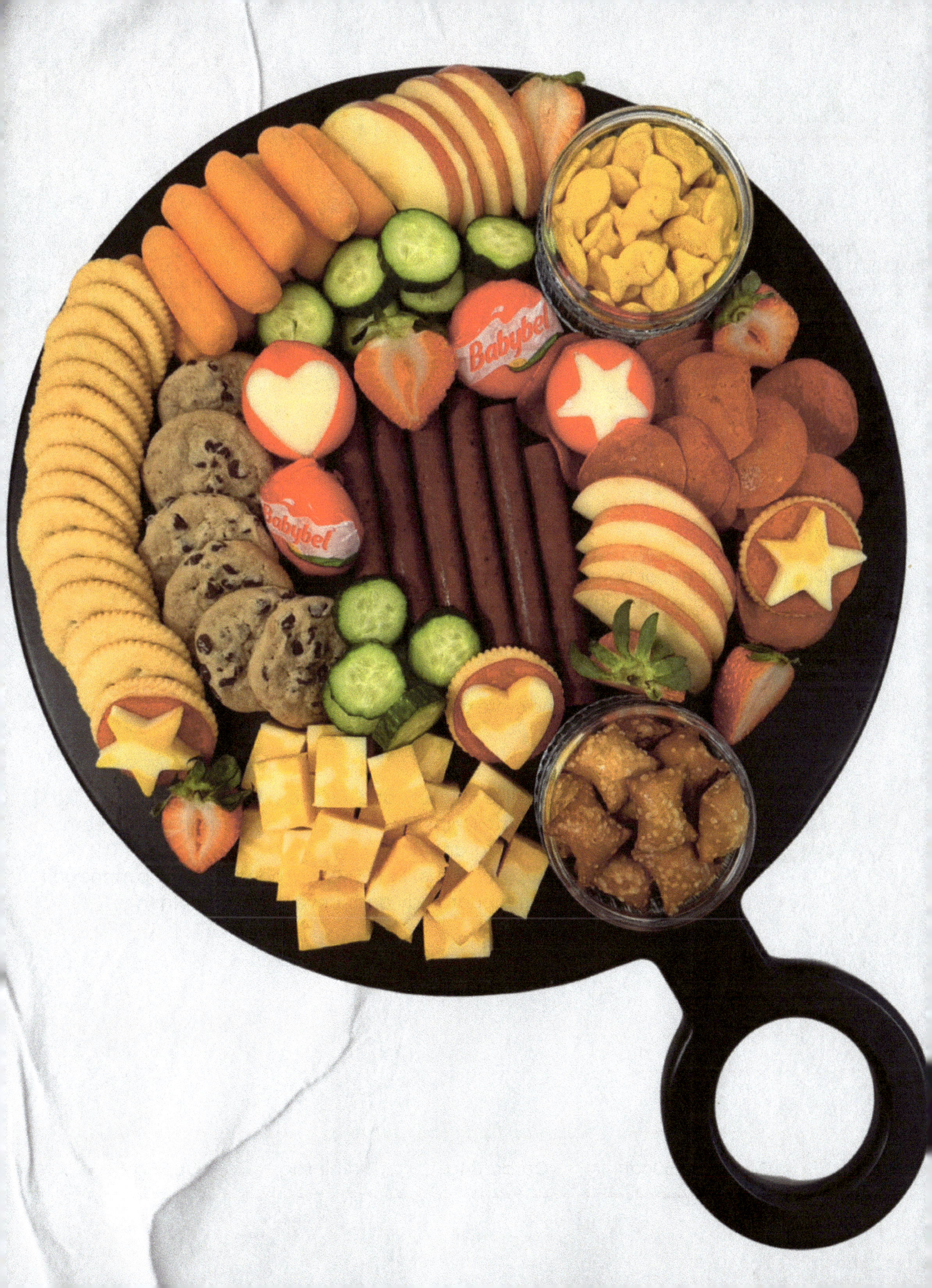
Babybel
Babybel

Junk Food Board

🍴 Preparation time
5 minutes

🛎 Serving
4

Ingredients:

- » 2 cups Skinny Pop popcorn
- » 2 cups Flaming Hot Cheetos
- » 1 pack Lay's Potato Chips
- » 8 mini size Snickers
- » 1 pack SOUR PATCH KIDS
- » 10 OREO cookies
- » 4 Twinkies
- » 1 cup M&MS

Instructions:

1. On a large platter or board, arrange the Skinny Pop popcorn, Flaming Hot Cheetos, and Lay's Potato Chips in separate sections.
2. Place the Snickers (fun-size), SOUR PATCH KIDS, OREO Cookies, and Twinkies in individual sections around the board.
3. Fill a small section with M&MS.
4. Serve immediately or cover and store at room temperature until ready to serve.

Tips

1. Balance sweet treats like Snickers and Twinkies with savory snacks like Cheetos and Lay's Potato Chips for a delightful mix. Group similar items together for a neat appearance.
2. Use small bowls or cups for items like M&Ms and popcorn to help manage portions. This keeps the board tidy and prevents overindulgence.

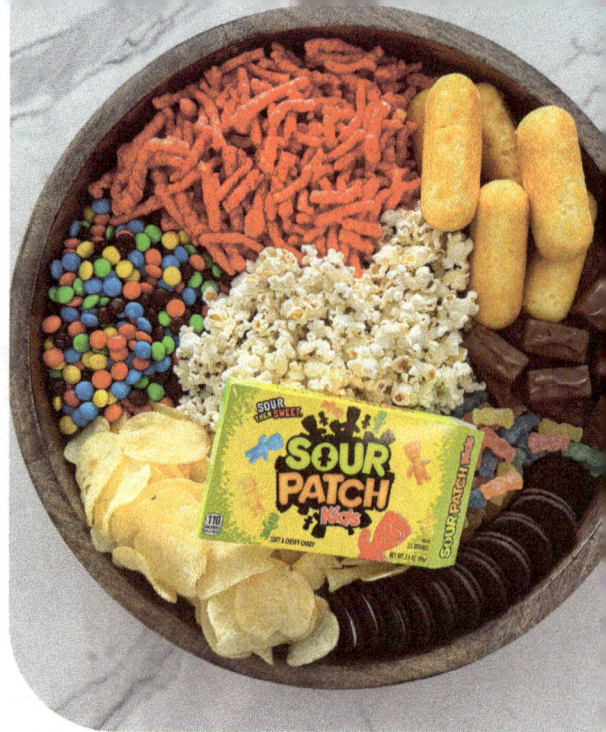

Nutrition facts (per serving)

| Calories: 750cal, | Carbs: 84g, | Protein: 6g, | Fat: 35g |

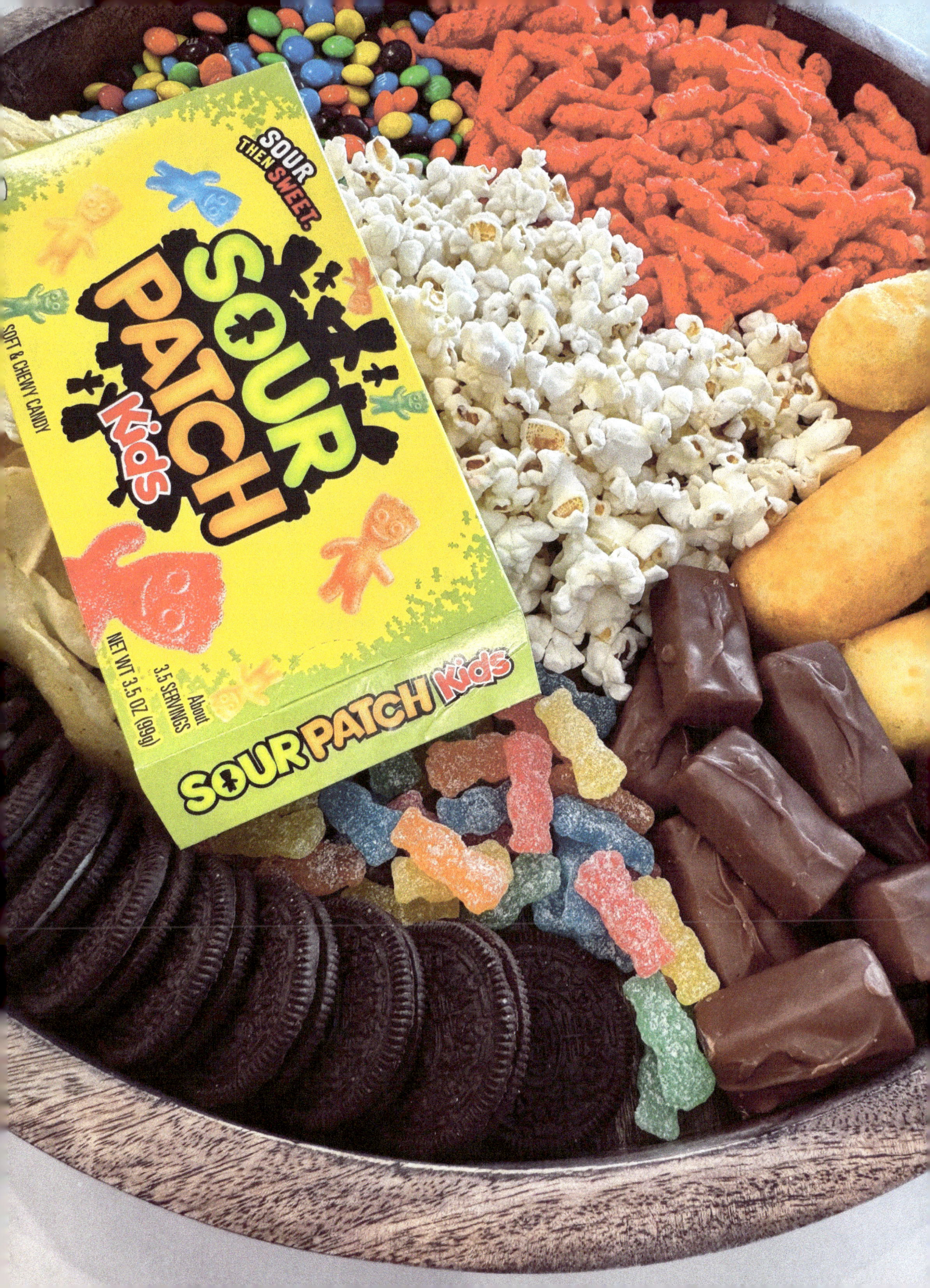

Classic Charcuterie Board

🍴 Preparation time 20 minutes   🔔 Serving 4

Ingredients:

- » 6 oz Columbus brand salami
- » 6 oz Italian dry salami log
- » 6 oz prosciutto
- » 4 oz creamy toscano
- » 5 oz Brie wedge
- » ½ cup candied pecans
- » ½ cup dried apricots
- » ½ cup marcona almonds
- » ½ cup castelvetrano olives
- » ½ cup cornichon pickles
- » 12 flatbread crackers
- » 5 strawberries
- » ½ cup spicy fig jam
- » Rosemary & sage garnish: a few sprigs for decoration

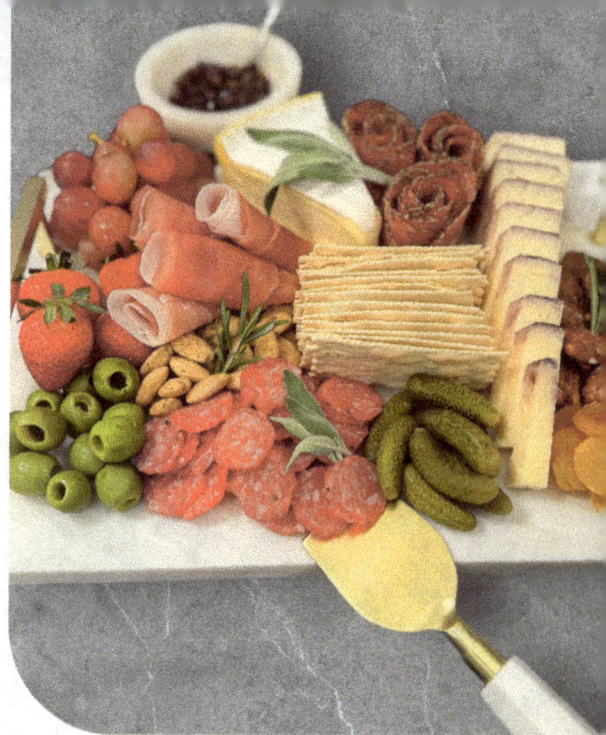

Instructions:

1. Firstly, slice the salami log and cube the Creamy Toscano cheese.
2. On a large platter or board, arrange the Columbus Salami, Italian Dry salami slices, and prosciutto in separate sections.
3. Place the Creamy Toscano cubes and Brie wedge on the board.
4. Arrange the candied pecans, dried apricots, Marcona almonds, Castelvetrano olives, and cornichon pickles in sections.
5. Position the flatbread crackers and strawberries around the board. Add a small bowl or section with the spicy fig jam.
6. Garnish with rosemary and sage sprigs for a decorative touch.
7. Serve immediately or cover and refrigerate until ready to serve.

Tips Include a mix of soft, creamy cheeses and firm, aged cheeses for texture variety. Add crunchy elements like nuts and pickles for an extra dimension.

Nutrition facts (per serving)

Calories: 600cal,	Carbs: 26g,	Protein: 22g,	Fat: 35g

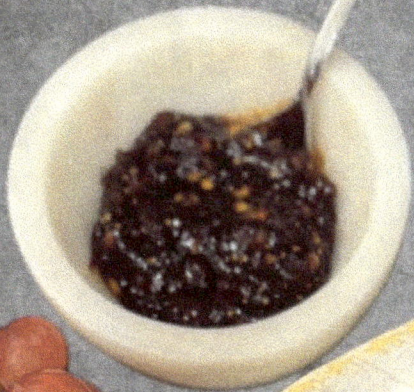

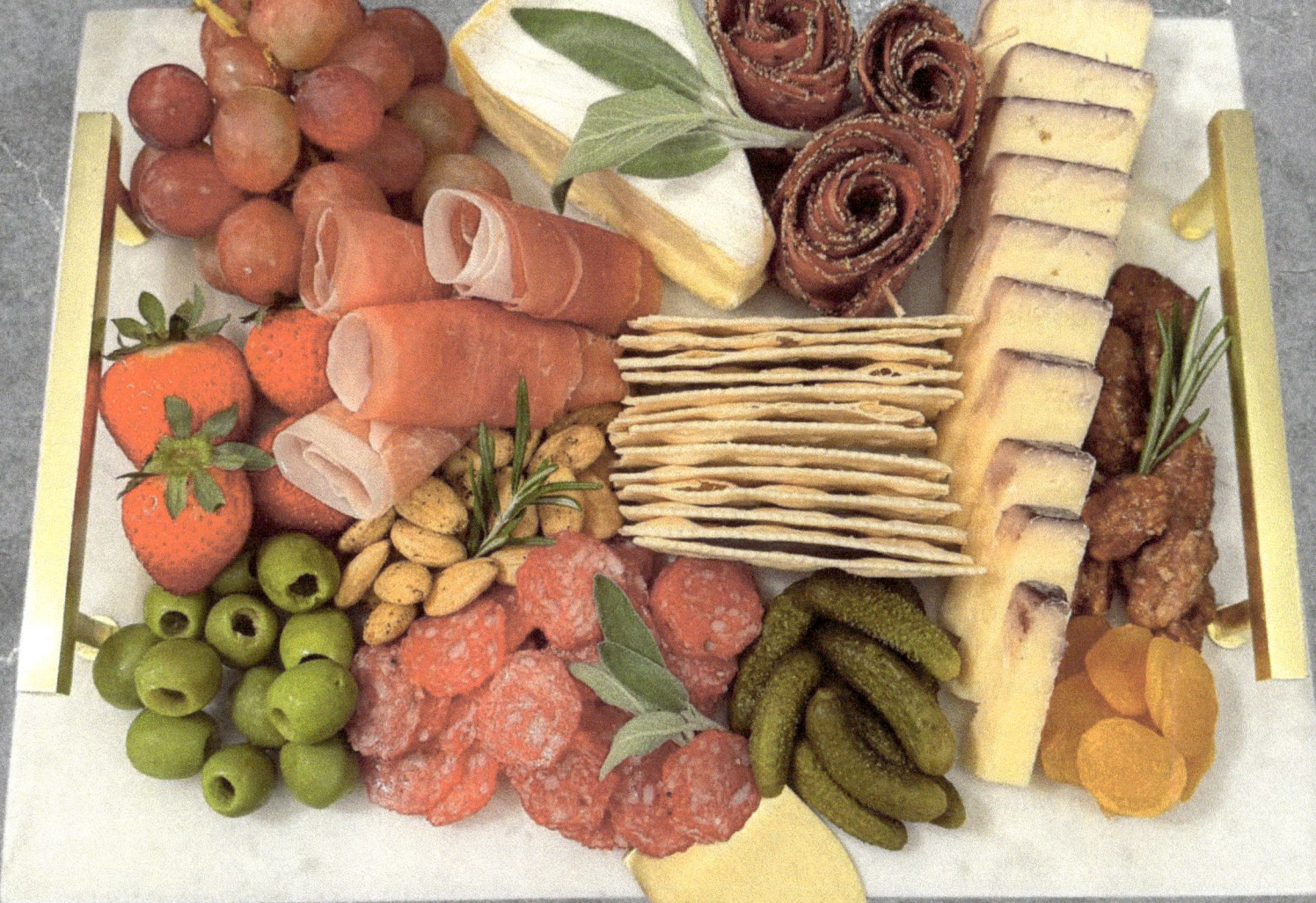

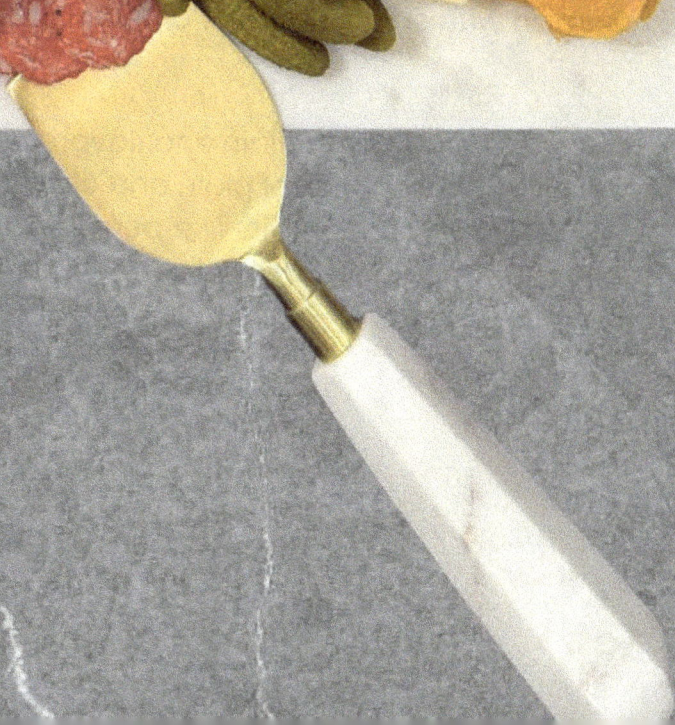

Brunch Board

🌸 Preparation time
15 minutes

🔔 Serving
3

Ingredients:

» 3 mini bagels (plain)
» 3 mini bagels (cinnamon raisin)
» 1 cup cream cheese
» 4 oz smoked salmon
» 1 cup each of strawberries, blueberries, and raspberries (total 15 oz)
» ½ small cubed cantaloupe
» ½ small pineapple
» 2 boiled eggs
» Dill for garnish: a few sprigs

Instructions:

1. Boil and peel the eggs, then halve them.
2. Cube the cantaloupe and pineapple.
3. Wash the berries and grapes.
4. On a large platter or board, arrange the mini bagels in one section.
5. Place the cream cheese in a small bowl or in dollops in between the board.
6. Arrange the smoked salmon near the bagels and cream cheese.
7. Place the halved boiled eggs in a section.
8. Arrange the berry trio, cantaloupe, pineapple, and green grapes in separate sections around the board.
9. Garnish with sprigs of dill for a decorative touch.

Tips

1. Add both plain and flavored cream cheeses to cater to different tastes. Use a mix of plain and cinnamon raisin mini bagels for variety.
2. Arrange fruits like berries and grapes around the board for color and balance. Use dill sprigs as a garnish to enhance the visual appeal.

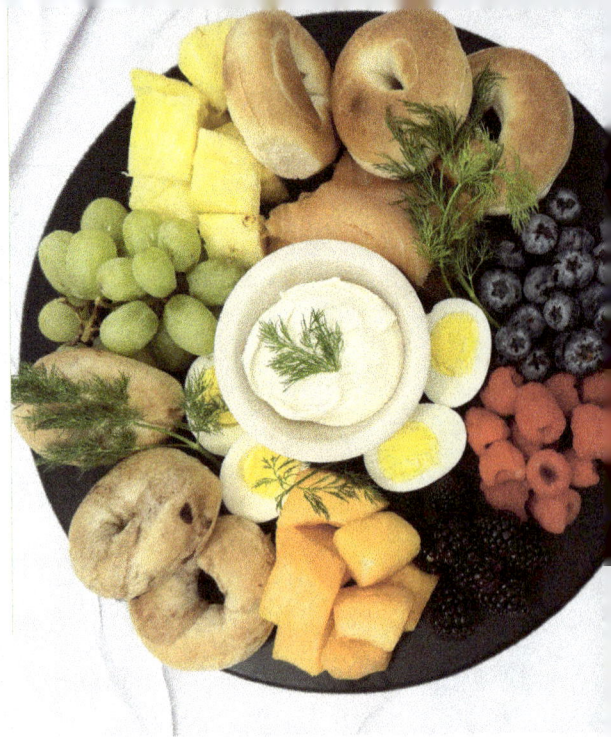

Nutrition facts (per serving)

Calories: 500cal,	Carbs: 50g,	Protein: 15g,	Fat: 20g

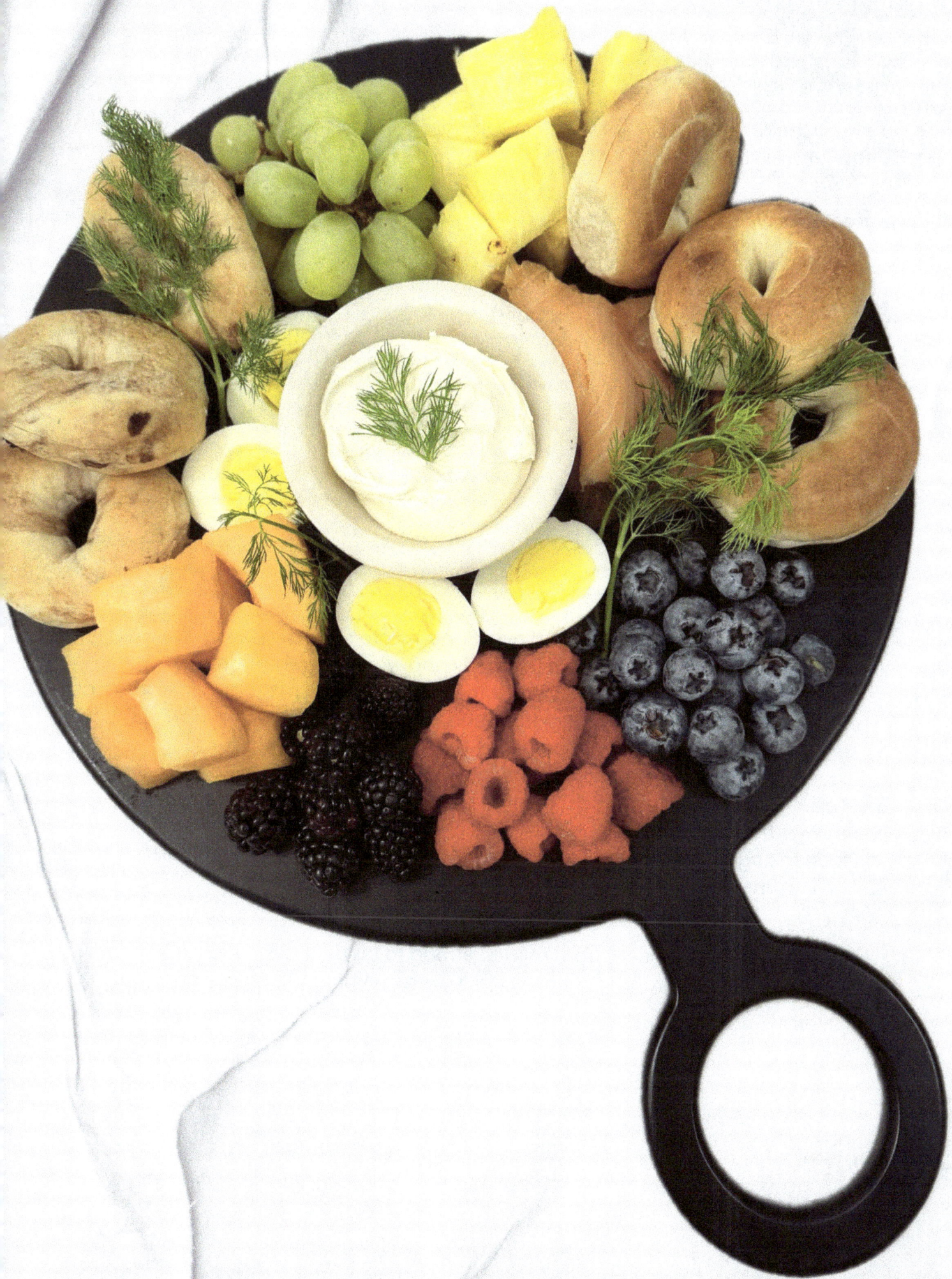

Cheese Board

Preparation time
5 minutes

Serving
4

Ingredients:

» 5 oz Brie wedge (soft, double or triple cream)
» 5 oz havarti dill (semi-soft)
» 4 oz fine herbs goat cheese (crumbly)
» 4 oz aged white cheddar (firm)
» 4 oz aged gouda (hard)
» 4 oz buttermilk blue (blue)
» ½ cup red grapes
» ¼ cup honey
» ½ cup marcona almonds
» 1 box fig & olive artisan crisps
» 1 baguette artisan baguette, sliced

Instructions:

1. Slice the aged white cheddar and aged gouda into small wedges.
2. Slice the artisan baguette into thin pieces and wash the red grapes.
3. On a large platter or board, arrange the Brie wedge, Havarti dill, fine herbs goat cheese, aged white cheddar, aged gouda, and Buttermilk Blue cheese in separate sections.
4. Place the red grapes around the cheeses.
5. Drizzle honey over a small section of the board or serve it in a small bowl.
6. Arrange the Marcona almonds near the cheeses.
7. Place the fig & olive artisan crisps and sliced baguette around the board.
8. Serve immediately or cover and refrigerate until ready to serve.

Tips
Arrange cheeses from mild to strong to guide the tasting experience. This prevents stronger cheeses from overwhelming the palate early on.

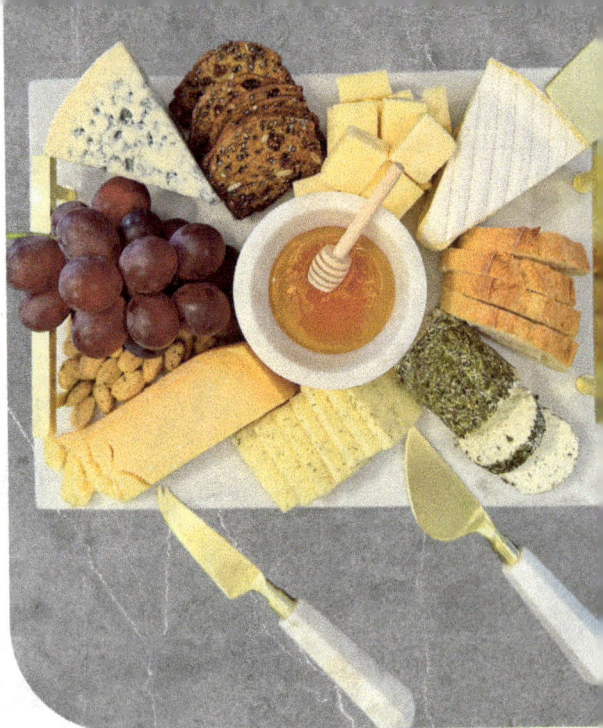

Nutrition facts (per serving)

Calories: 570cal,   Carbs: 45g,   Protein: 20g,   Fat: 30g

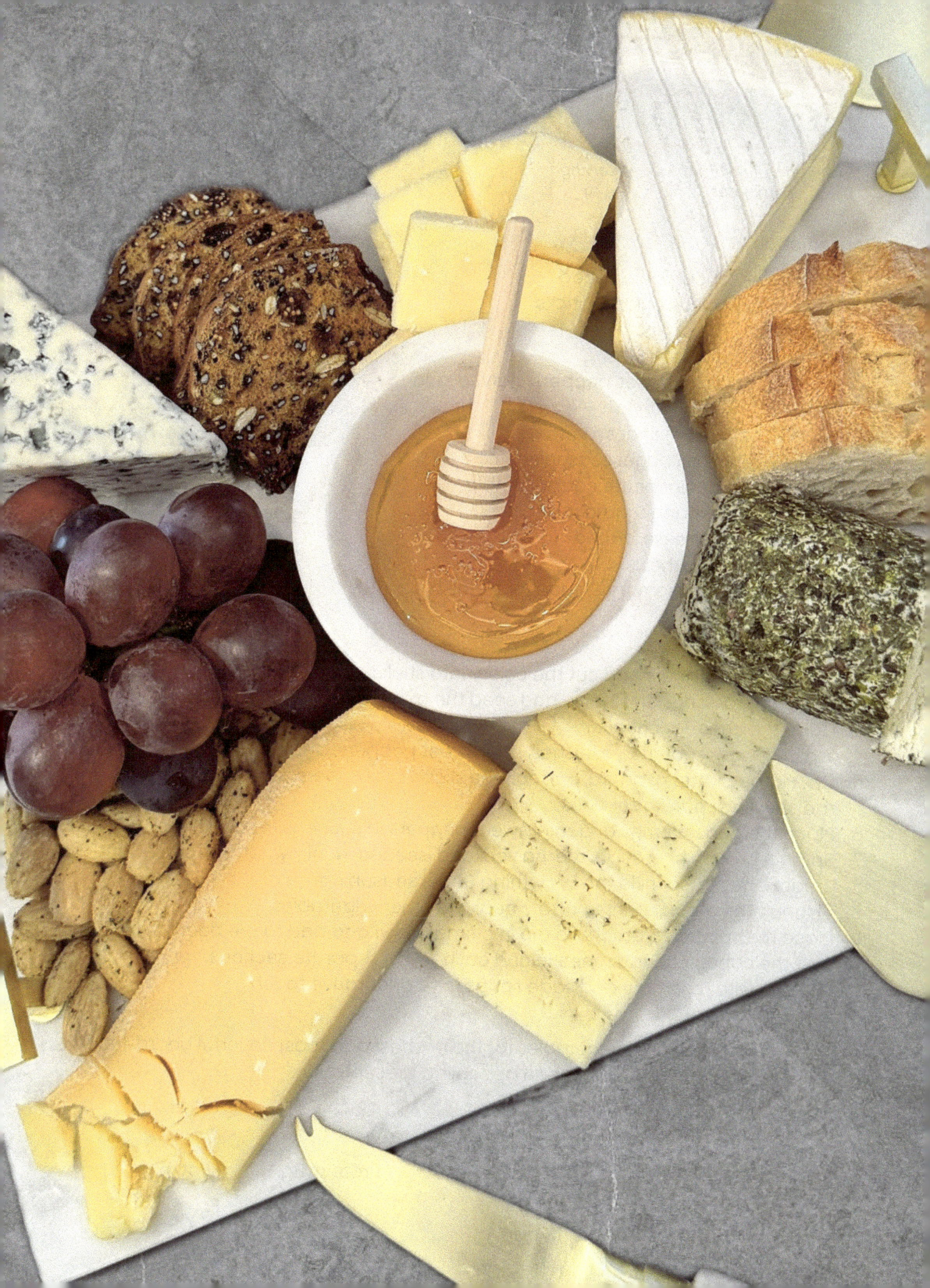

Vegetarian Board

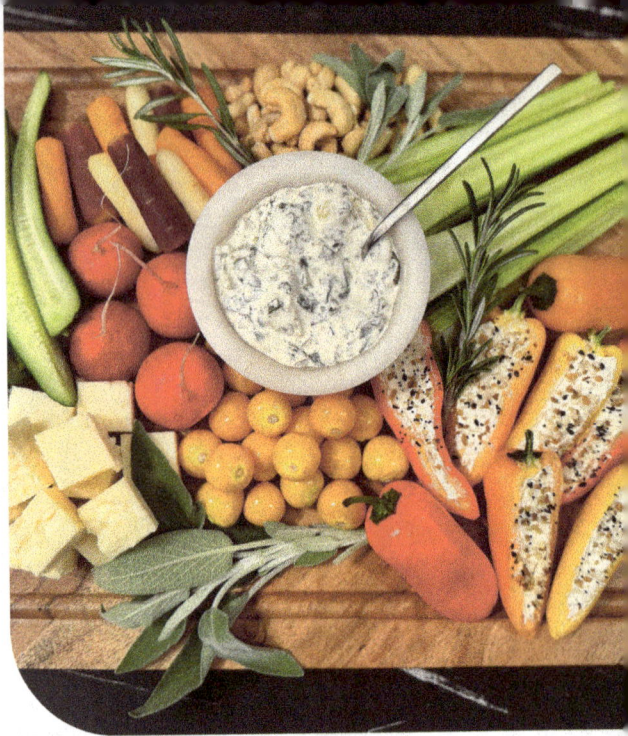

% Preparation time
15 minutes

🍽 Serving
6

Ingredients:

» 1 cup (5 oz) cucumbers, sliced
» 1 cup (5 oz) celery, cut into sticks
» 1 cup (4 oz) radishes, halved
» 1 cup (6 oz) gooseberries
» 1 cup (5 oz) mini sweet peppers, halved and seeded
» 1 cup (8 oz) cream cheese spread
» 2 tbsp everything bagel seasoning
» 1 cup (5 oz) tricolor petite carrots, whole
» 1 cup (8 oz) spinach & artichoke dip
» 4 oz cheddar cheese, cubed
» 1/2 cup (2 oz) cashews
» A few sprigs of rosemary & sage for garnish

Instructions:

1. Slice the cucumbers and cut the celery into sticks.
2. Halve the radishes also halve and seed the mini sweet peppers.
3. Cube the cheddar cheese.
4. Wash the gooseberries, radishes, mini sweet peppers, and petite carrots.
5. On a large platter or board, arrange the sliced cucumbers, celery sticks, and halved radishes in separate sections.
6. Place the gooseberries and mini sweet peppers in sections around the board.
7. Spread cream cheese in the halved and seeded mini sweet peppers. Over the cream cheese, sprinkle the Everything Bagel seasoning.
8. Arrange the tricolor petite carrots near the other vegetables.
9. Place the spinach & artichoke dip in a small bowl and add to the board.
10. Add the cubed cheddar cheese and cashews in separate sections.
11. Garnish with rosemary and sage sprigs for a decorative touch.

Tips Use seasonal vegetables for the freshest and most flavorful board. Include a variety of colors for an appealing presentation.

Nutrition facts (per serving)

| Calories: 220cal, | Carbs: 18g, | Protein: 8g, | Fat: 15g |

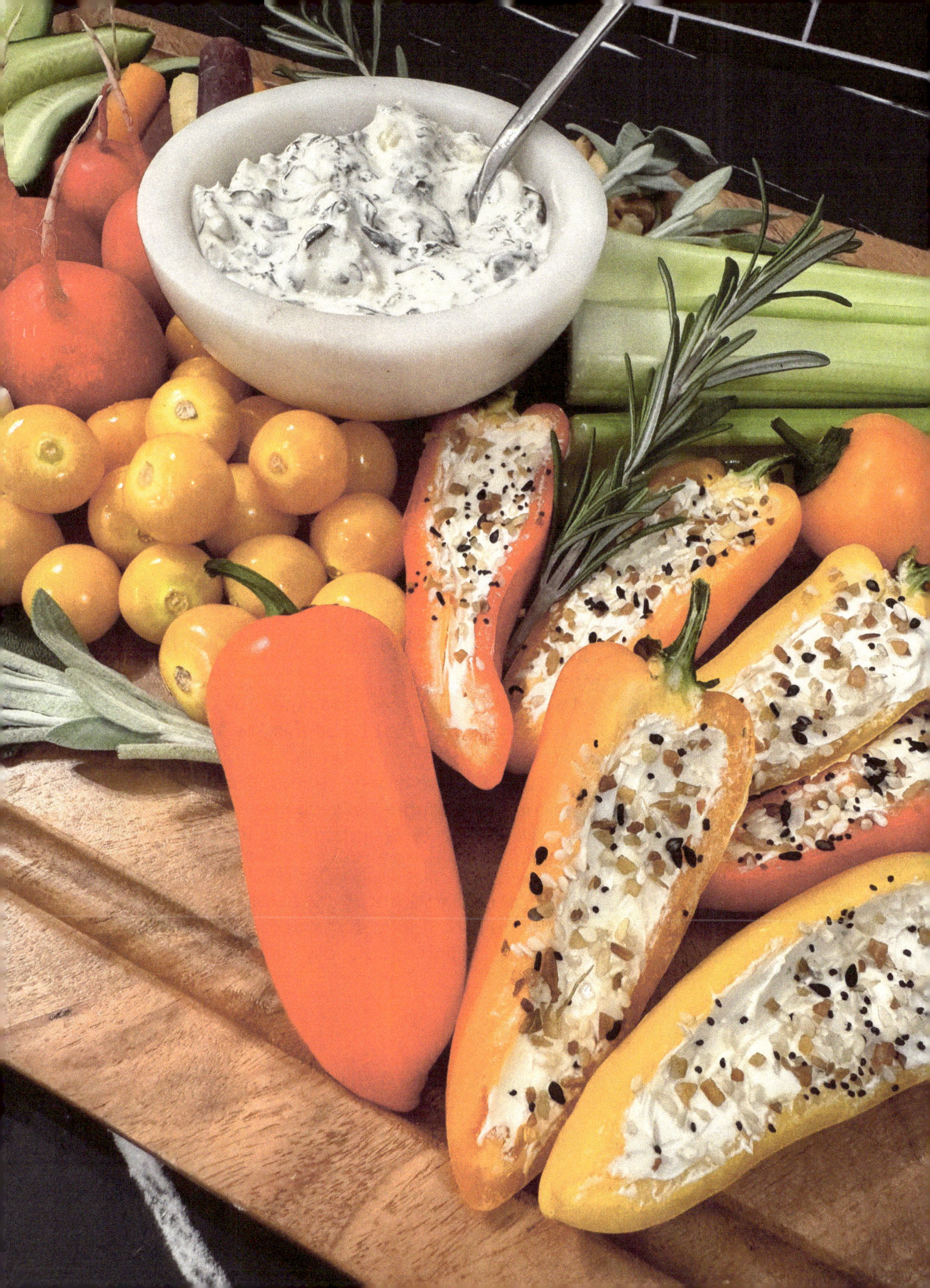

Fruit Board

🌸 Preparation time
20 minutes

🔔 Serving
6

Ingredients:

» 5 strawberries, halved
» 2 kiwis, peeled and sliced
» 1 red dragon fruit, peeled and cubed
» ½ cup blackberries
» 1 cup pineapple
» 1 orange, peeled and segmented
» 1 cup watermelon in slices
» 1 cup green grapes
» 1 cup cream cheese fruit dip

Instructions:

1. Halve the strawberries also peel and slice the kiwis.
2. Peel and cube the red dragon fruit.
3. Slice the pineapple and watermelon
4. Peel and segment the oranges.
5. Wash the strawberries, blackberries, green grapes, and other fruits.
6. On a large platter or board, arrange the halved strawberries, kiwi slices, and cubed red dragon fruit in separate sections.
7. Place the blackberries, pineapple cubes, and orange segments around the board.
8. Arrange the watermelon cubes and green grapes in sections.
9. Place the cream cheese fruit dip in a small bowl and add it to the board.

Tips
Pre-cut all fruits for ease of serving. Ensure they are bite-sized and easy to pick up and arrange the fruits by contrasting colors for a vibrant display. This makes the board more inviting and visually striking.

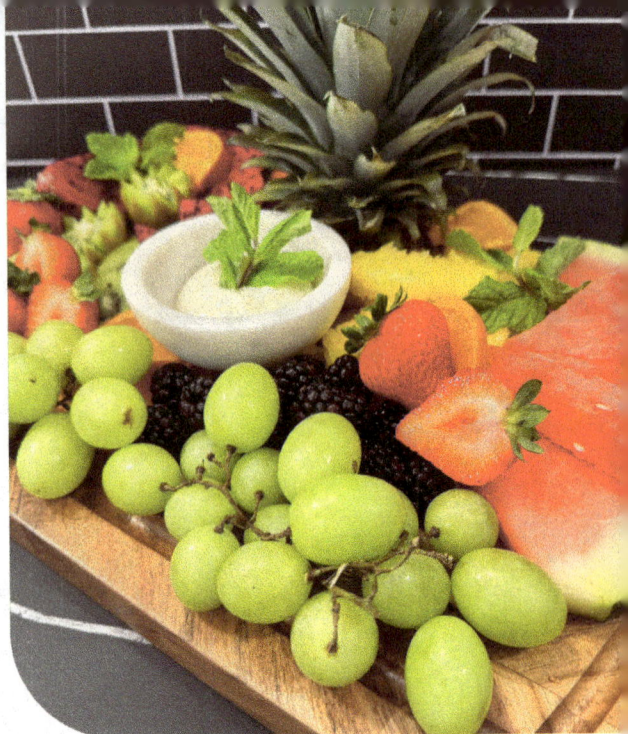

Nutrition facts (per serving)

Calories: 180cal,   Carbs: 30g,   Protein: 2g,   Fat: 6g

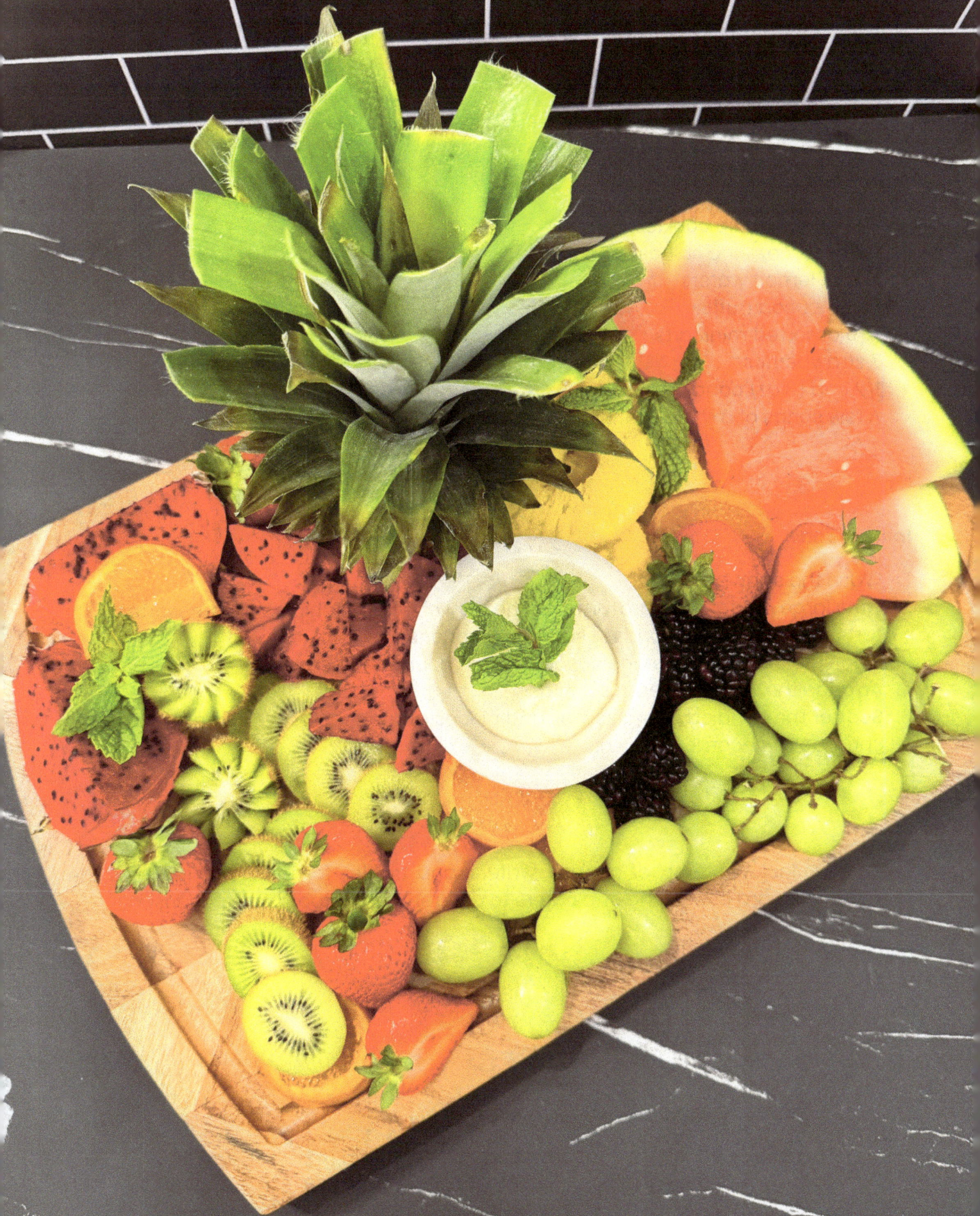

Dessert Board

🌸 Preparation time
5 minutes

🛎 Serving
4

Ingredients:

» 8 chocolate chip cookies
» 1/2 cup (2 oz) sea salt almonds
» 1 pack lemon wafers
» 1 cup cocoa truffles
» 4-6 assorted mini tarts
» 7 strawberries
» 1/2 cup (3 oz) candied oranges
» A few sprigs of mint for garnish

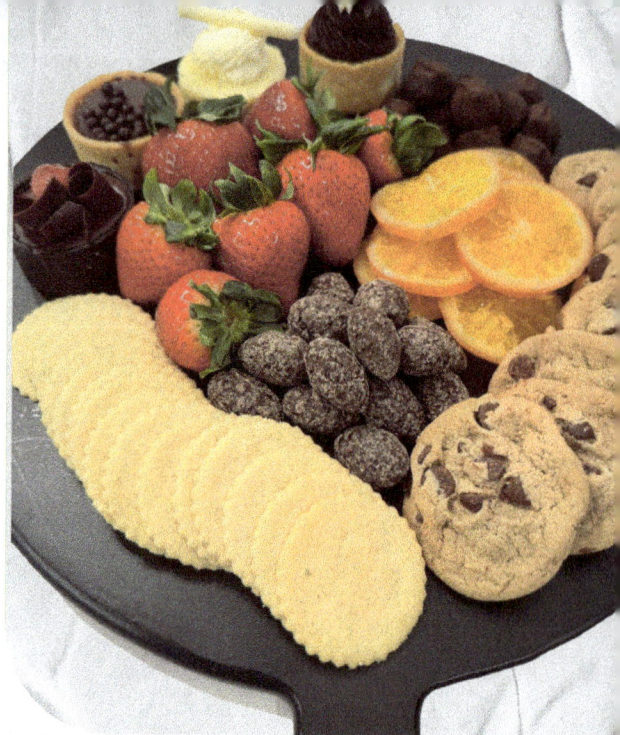

Instructions:

1. Wash the strawberries.
2. On a large platter or board, arrange the mini chocolate chip cookies, assorted mini tarts, and sea salt almonds in separate sections.
3. Place the lemon wafers and cocoa truffles around the board.
4. Arrange the strawberries in sections.
5. Scatter the candied orange slices and pieces around the board. Garnish with mint sprigs for a decorative touch.

Tips Include a mix of cookies, wafers, and truffles for variety. This keeps the board interesting and caters to different sweet tooth preferences.

Nutrition facts (per serving)

Calories: 500cal,   Carbs: 60g,   Protein: 7g,   Fat: 25g

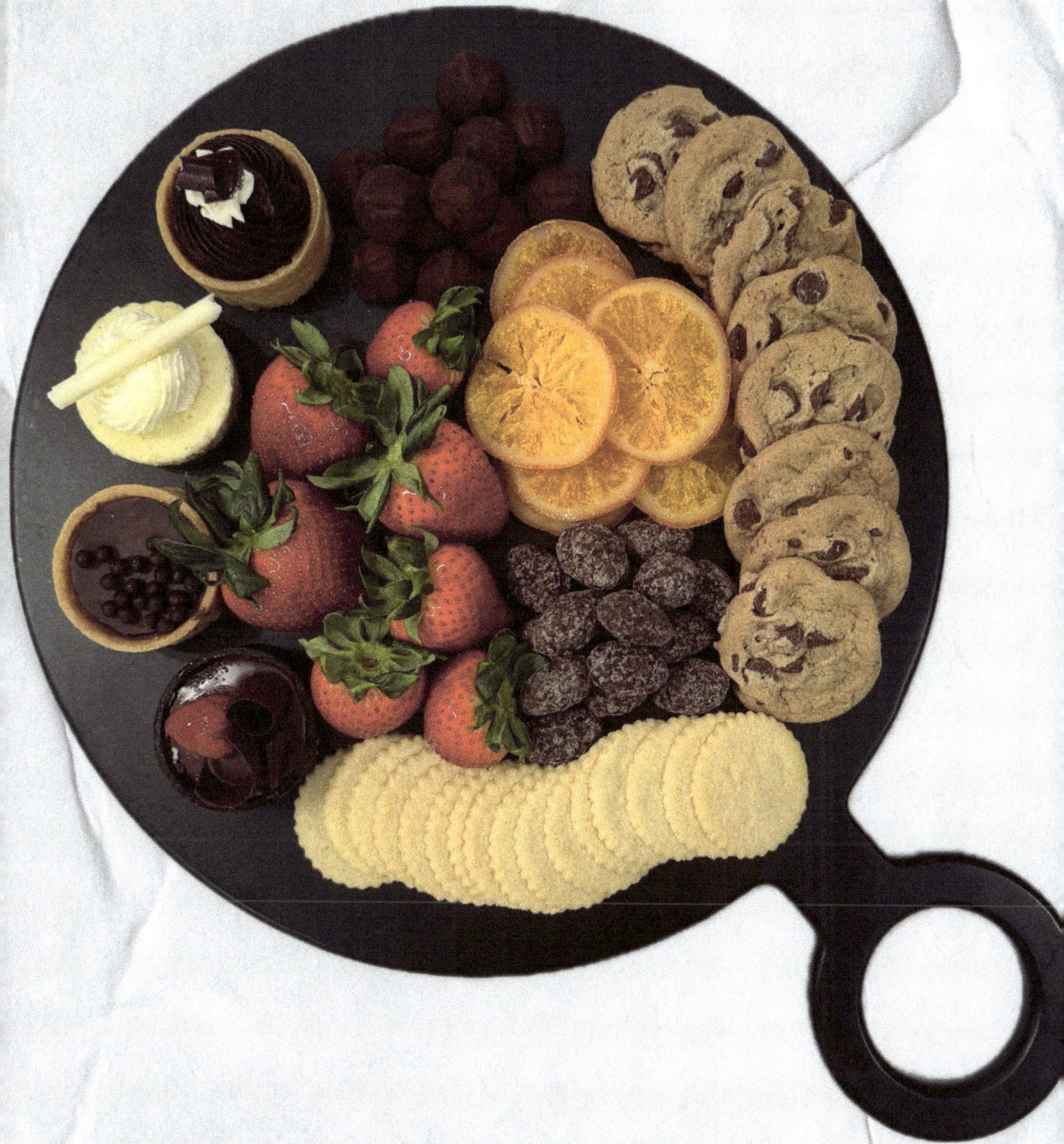

Individual Servings

Preparation time
10 minutes

Serving
1

Ingredients:

- » 2 tbsp marcona almonds
- » 2 tbsp candied pecans
- » 2 tbsp dried cranberries
- » 2 oz salami nuggets
- » 2 oz Brie cheese bites
- » 2 oz white cheddar cheese, cubed
- » 4 almond stuffed olives
- » 1 sprig rosemary garnish

Instructions:

1. Cube the white cheddar cheese.
2. In a small bowl, arrange the Marcona almonds, candied pecans, and dried cranberries in separate sections.
3. Place the salami nuggets, Brie cheese bites, and white cheddar cheese cubes around the plate.
4. Add the almond stuffed olives.
5. Garnish with a sprig of rosemary for a decorative touch.

Tips Use small cups or bowls for individual servings to keep the board tidy and manageable. This also ensures everyone gets an equal share.

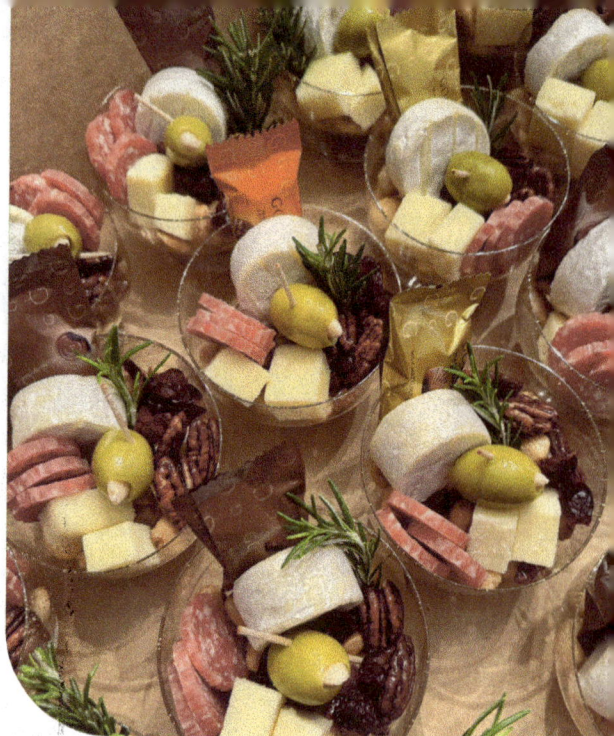

Nutrition facts (per serving)

Calories: 480cal,	Carbs: 22g,	Protein: 24g,	Fat: 40g

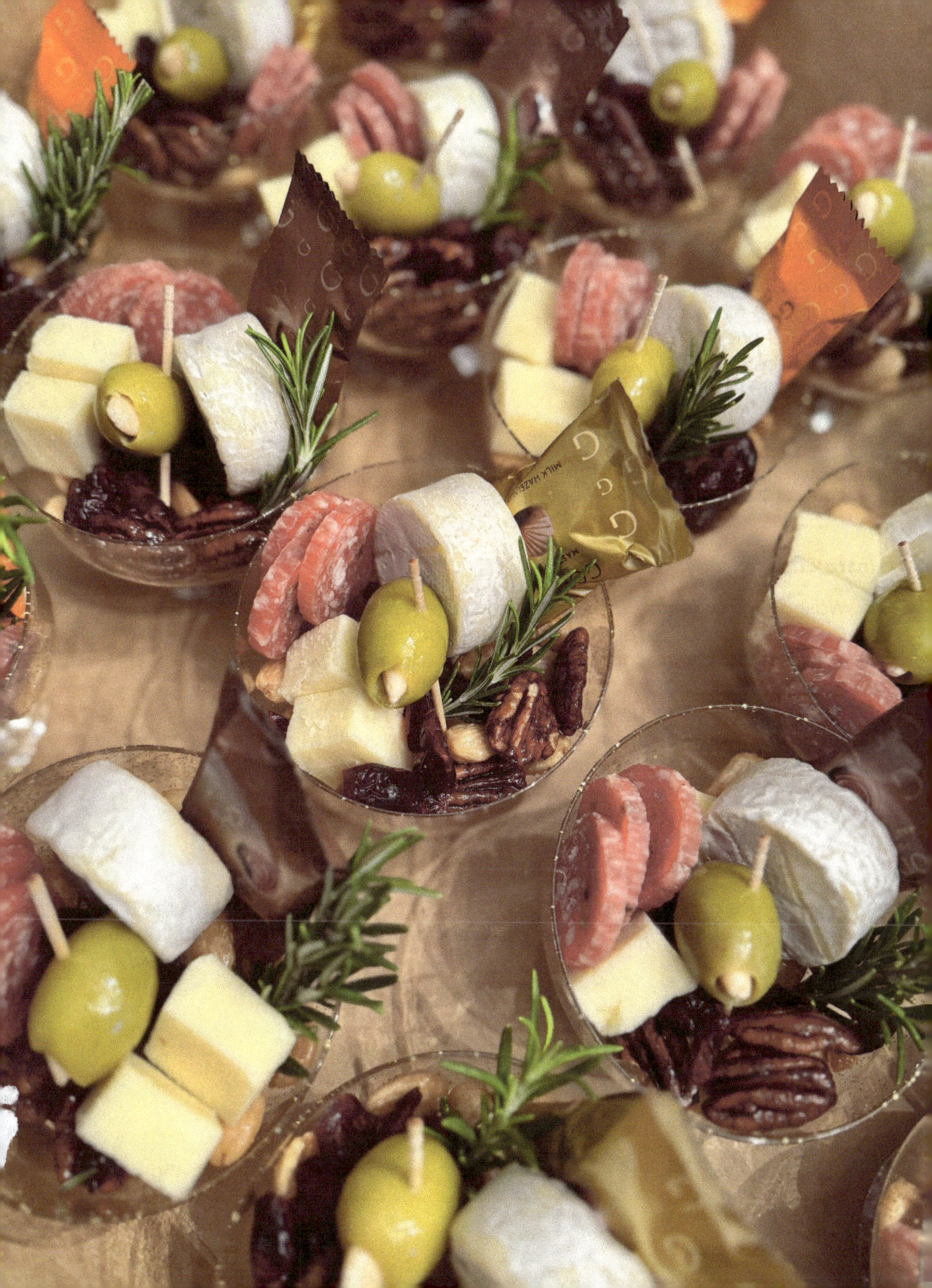

"Brie Mine" Love Board

Preparation time	Serving
5 minutes	4

Ingredients:

- » 1 round Brie cheese with a heart-shaped cutout
- » 1 cup fig & olive crackers
- » 1/4 cup honey
- » 7 strawberries
- » 1 cup (4 oz) raspberries
- » 1 cup (5 oz) red grapes
- » 6 raspberry macarons
- » 1/2 cup dark chocolate sea salt caramels
- » 1 cup cracker-cut cheddar cheese

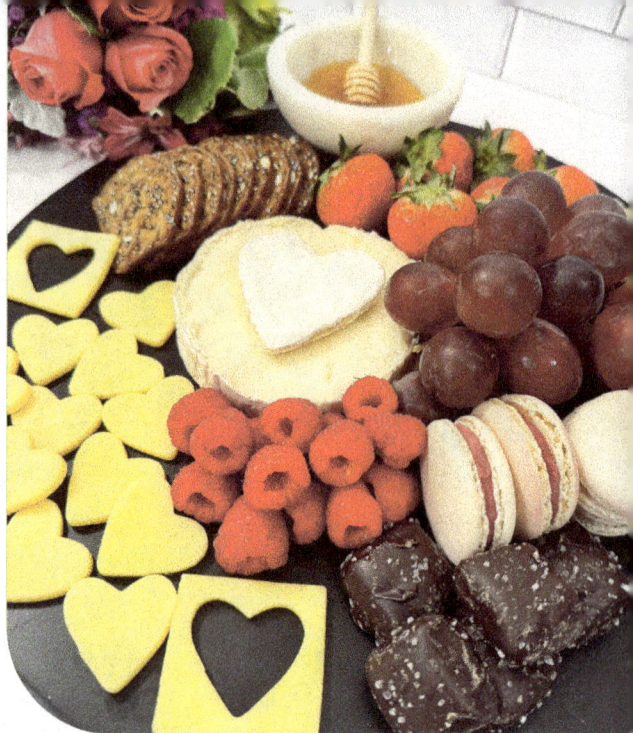

Instructions:

1. Wash the strawberries, raspberries, and red grapes.
2. Cut a heart shape out of the center of the Brie cheese round.
3. Place the Brie cheese round in the center of a large platter or board.
4. Arrange the Fig & Olive crackers around the Brie cheese.
5. Place the honey in a ramekin with a honey dipper near the Brie.
6. Arrange the strawberries, raspberries, and red grapes in sections around the board.
7. Place the raspberry macarons and dark chocolate sea salt caramels around the board.
8. Arrange the cracker-cut cheddar cheese in a section near the Brie.

Tips
Use a small cookie cutter to create a heart-shaped cutout in the Brie for a romantic touch. This adds a special and personal element to the board.

Nutrition facts (per serving)

Calories: 600cal,	Carbs: 50g,	Protein: 20g,	Fat: 45g

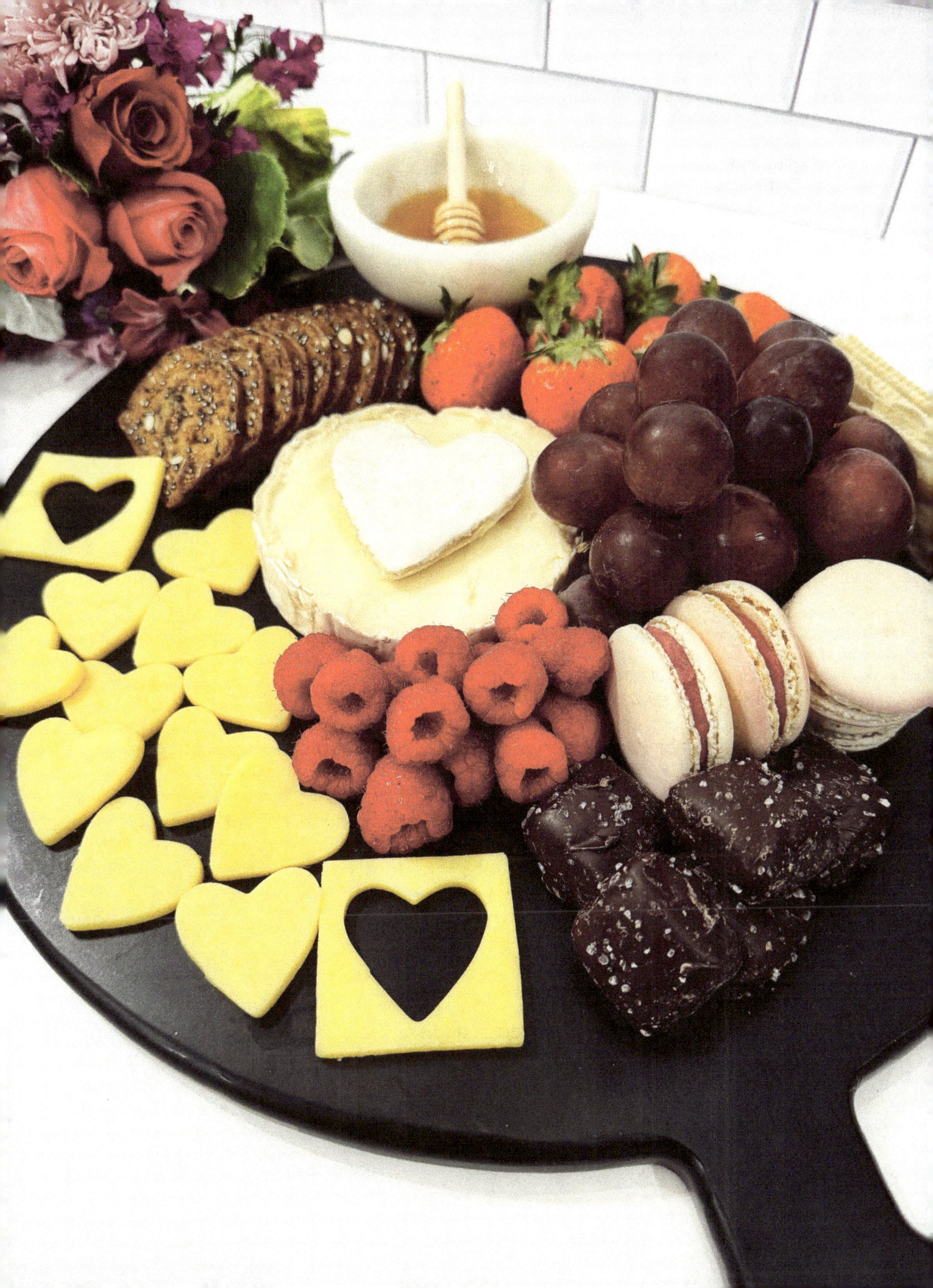

Bloody Mary Board

🌸 Preparation time
15 minutes

🛎 Serving
6

Ingredients:

- » 1 cup vodka
- » 2 cups tomato juice
- » 2 stalks celery, cut into sticks
- » 2 lemons or limes, cut into wedges
- » 1/2 cup cheese stuffed olives
- » 1/2 cup cornichons
- » 1/2 cup pepperoncini peppers
- » 1/2 cup pappadew peppers
- » 1/2 cup pepperjack cheese, cubed
- » 4 slices bacon, cooked
- » 4 sausage sticks
- » 1/2 cup cheddar cheese, cubed
- » 1 bottle (5 oz) Tabasco sauce
- » 1 cup mini sweet peppers, halved

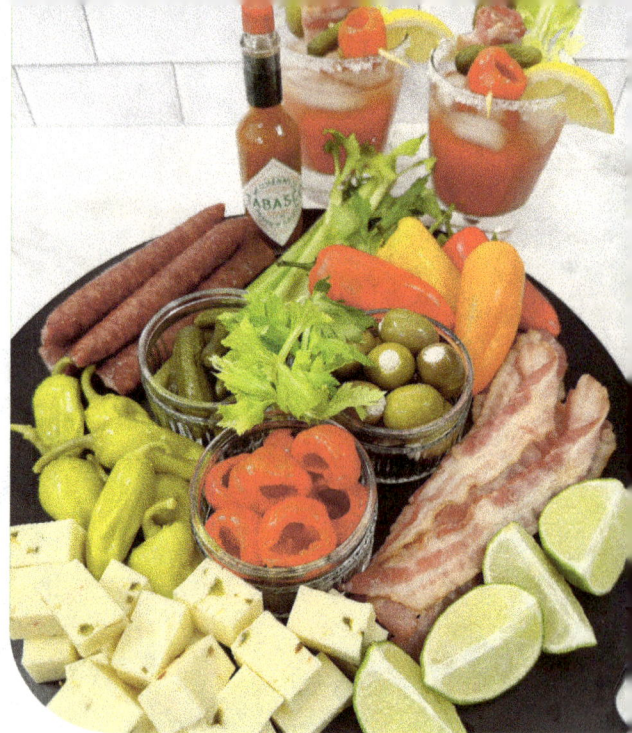

Instructions:

1. Cook the bacon until crispy and let it cool.
2. Cut the celery into sticks and cut the lemons or limes into wedges.
3. Cube the pepperjack cheese and cheddar cheese.
4. On a large platter or board, arrange the vodka and tomato juice in small carafes or glasses.
5. Place the celery sticks, lemon or lime wedges, cheese stuffed olives, cornichons, pepperoncini peppers, and pappadew peppers in separate sections around the board.
6. Arrange the pepperjack cheese cubes, cheddar cheese cubes, bacon slices, sausage sticks, and halved mini sweet peppers around the board.
7. Place the Tabasco sauce bottle in the center or near the tomato juice for easy access.

Tips

1. Use cocktail skewers to arrange items like olives, peppers, and cheese for easy handling. This adds a fun and practical element to the board.
2. Serve with a varitey of garnishes like celery and lemon wedges for customization.

Nutrition facts (per serving)

Calories: 550cal,	Carbs: 30g,	Protein: 25g,	Fat: 40g

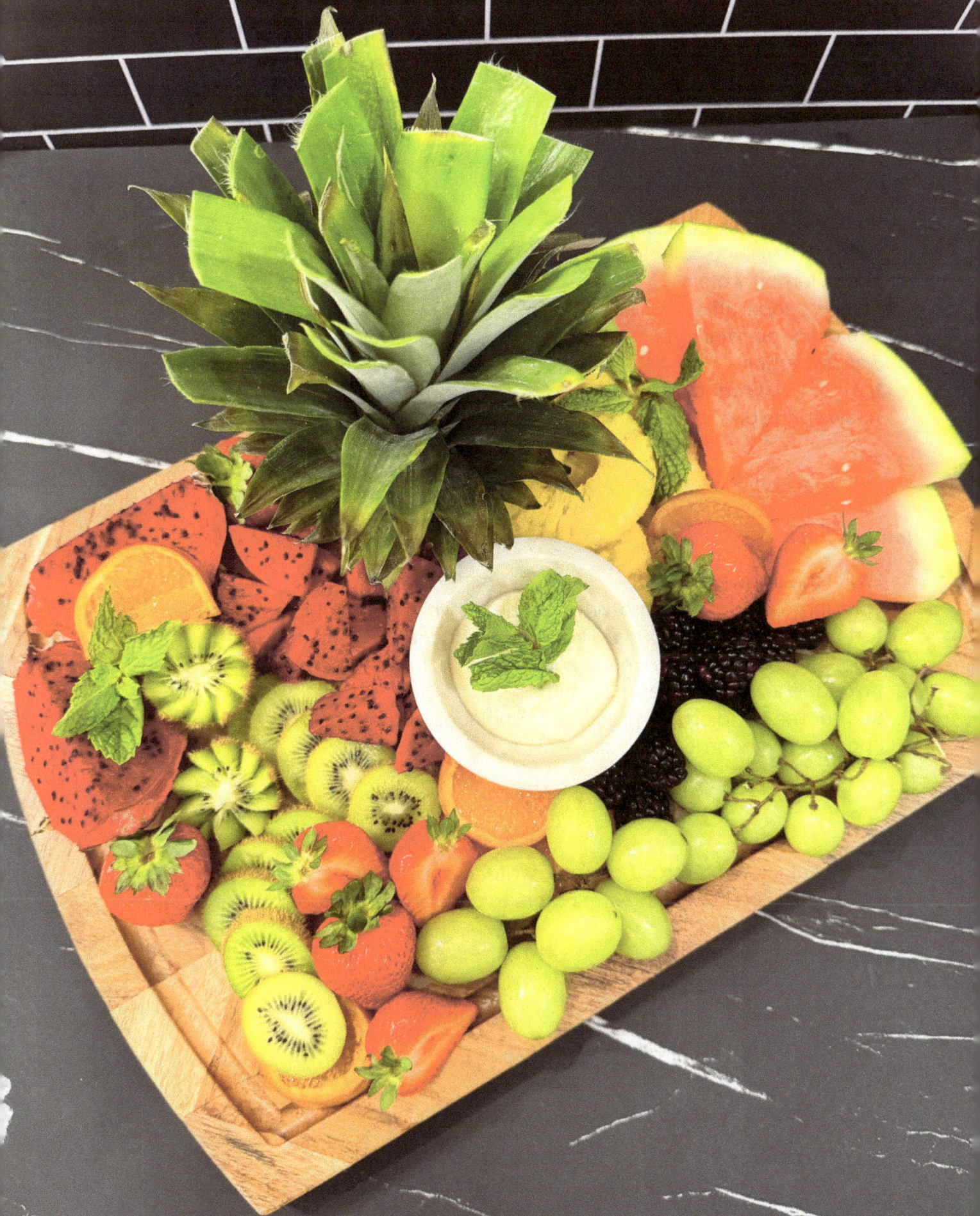

Dessert Board

%% Preparation time
5 minutes

🛎 Serving
4

Ingredients:

» 8 chocolate chip cookies
» 1/2 cup (2 oz) sea salt almonds
» 1 pack lemon wafers
» 1 cup cocoa truffles
» 4-6 assorted mini tarts
» 7 strawberries
» 1/2 cup (3 oz) candied oranges
» A few sprigs of mint for garnish

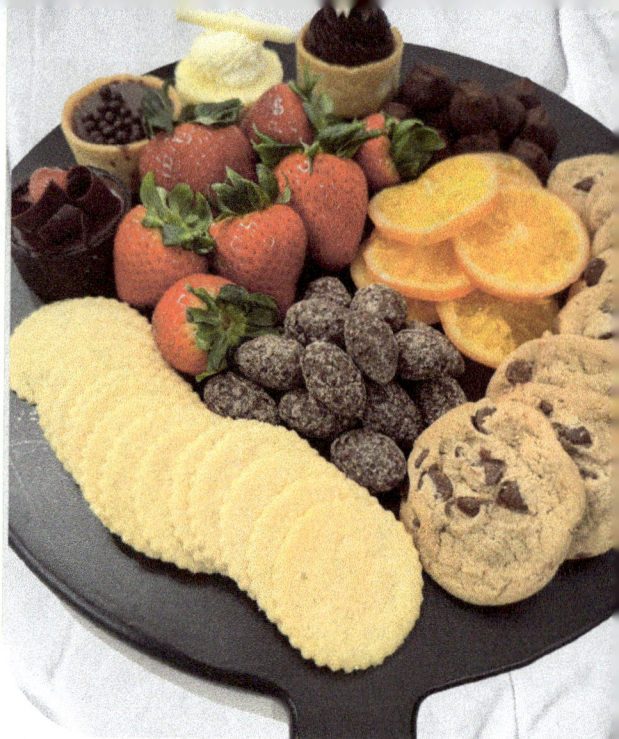

Instructions:

1. Wash the strawberries.
2. On a large platter or board, arrange the mini chocolate chip cookies, assorted mini tarts, and sea salt almonds in separate sections.
3. Place the lemon wafers and cocoa truffles around the board.
4. Arrange the strawberries in sections.
5. Scatter the candied orange slices and pieces around the board. Garnish with mint sprigs for a decorative touch.

Tips Include a mix of cookies, wafers, and truffles for variety. This keeps the board interesting and caters to different sweet tooth preferences.

Nutrition facts (per serving)

Calories: 500cal,   Carbs: 60g,   Protein: 7g,   Fat: 25g

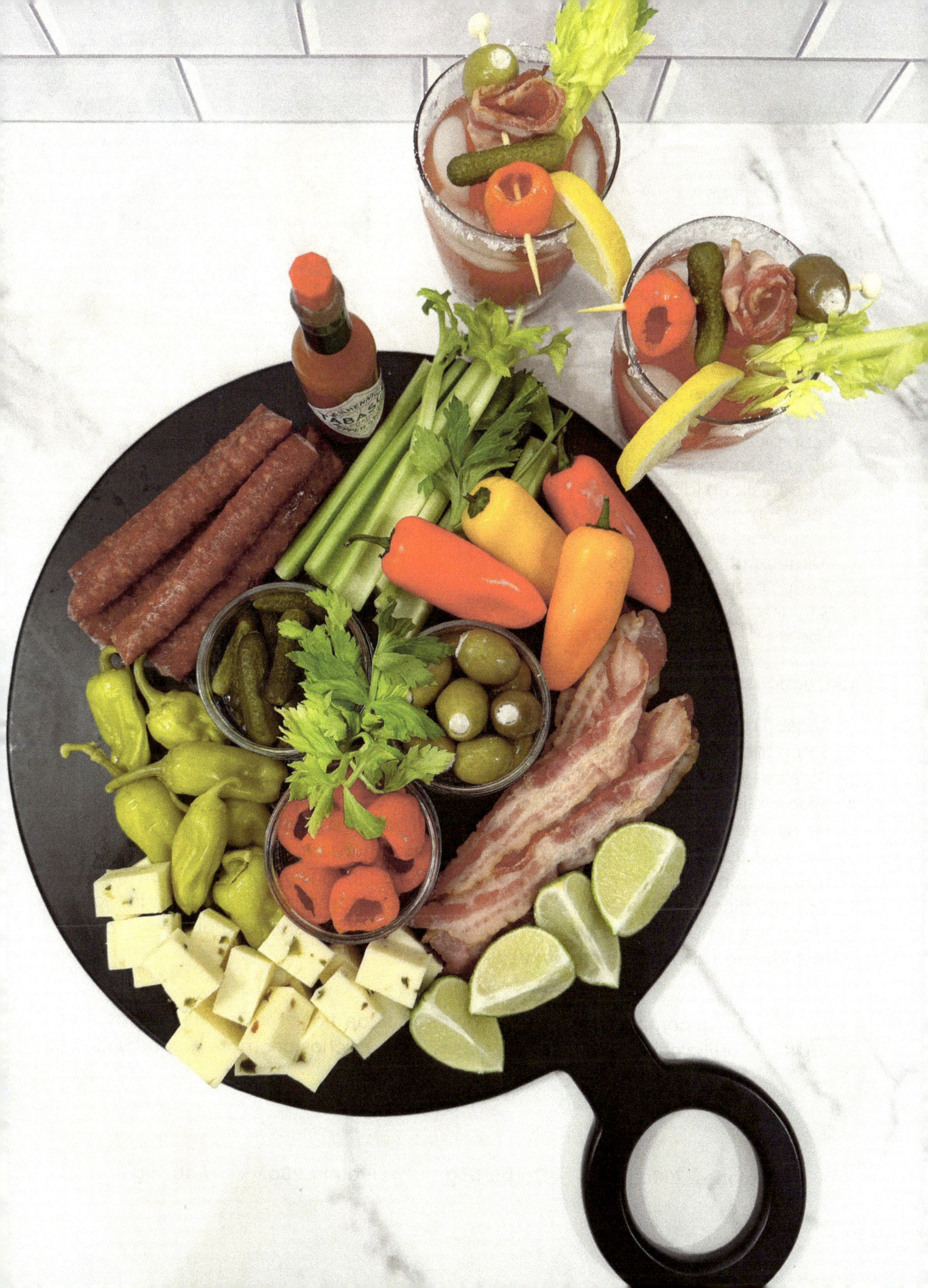

Taco Board

Preparation time 20 minutes	**Serving** 6

Ingredients:

» 1 lb seasoned and cooked ground beef
» 2 cups shredded lettuce
» 1 cup Mexican blend cheese, shredded
» 1 cup roasted corn (or elote)
» 1 cup sour cream
» 1 cup fresh guacamole
» 1 cup pico de gallo
» 1/2 cup diced white onions
» 1/4 cup sliced jalapeno
» 1 cup tomatoes, diced
» 1 avocado, sliced
» 2 limes, cut into wedges
» 2 cups corn tortilla chips
» 8 flour tortillas
» 1 bottle (5 oz) tabasco sauce

Instructions:

1. Season and cook the ground beef until fully cooked.
2. Shred the lettuce and mexican blend cheese.
3. Dice the white onions and tomatoes.
4. Slice the jalapeno and avocado and cut the limes into wedges.
5. On a large board or platter, place the ground beef in a bowl or section in the center.
6. Arrange the shredded lettuce, Mexican blend cheese, roasted corn, sour cream, fresh guacamole, and pico de gallo in separate sections around the beef.
7. Add the diced white onions, sliced jalapeno, diced tomatoes, and avocado slices.
8. Place the lime wedges, corn tortilla chips, and flour tortillas around the board. Include the Tabasco sauce for easy access.

Tips

To accommodate varying tastes, include flour tortillas as well as corn tortilla chips. This allows guests to have nachos or create tacos. Use fresh toppings as well.

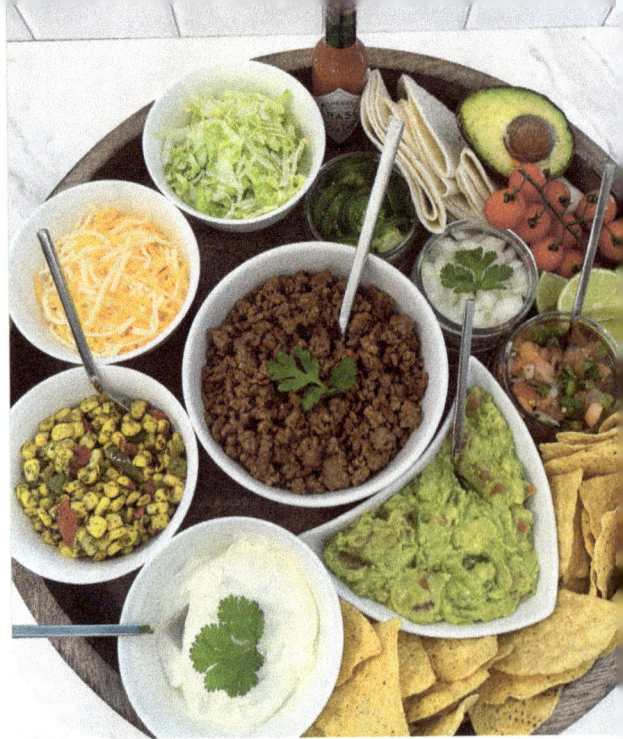

Nutrition facts (per serving)

Calories: 700cals,   Carbs: 55g,   Protein: 28g,   Fat: 45g

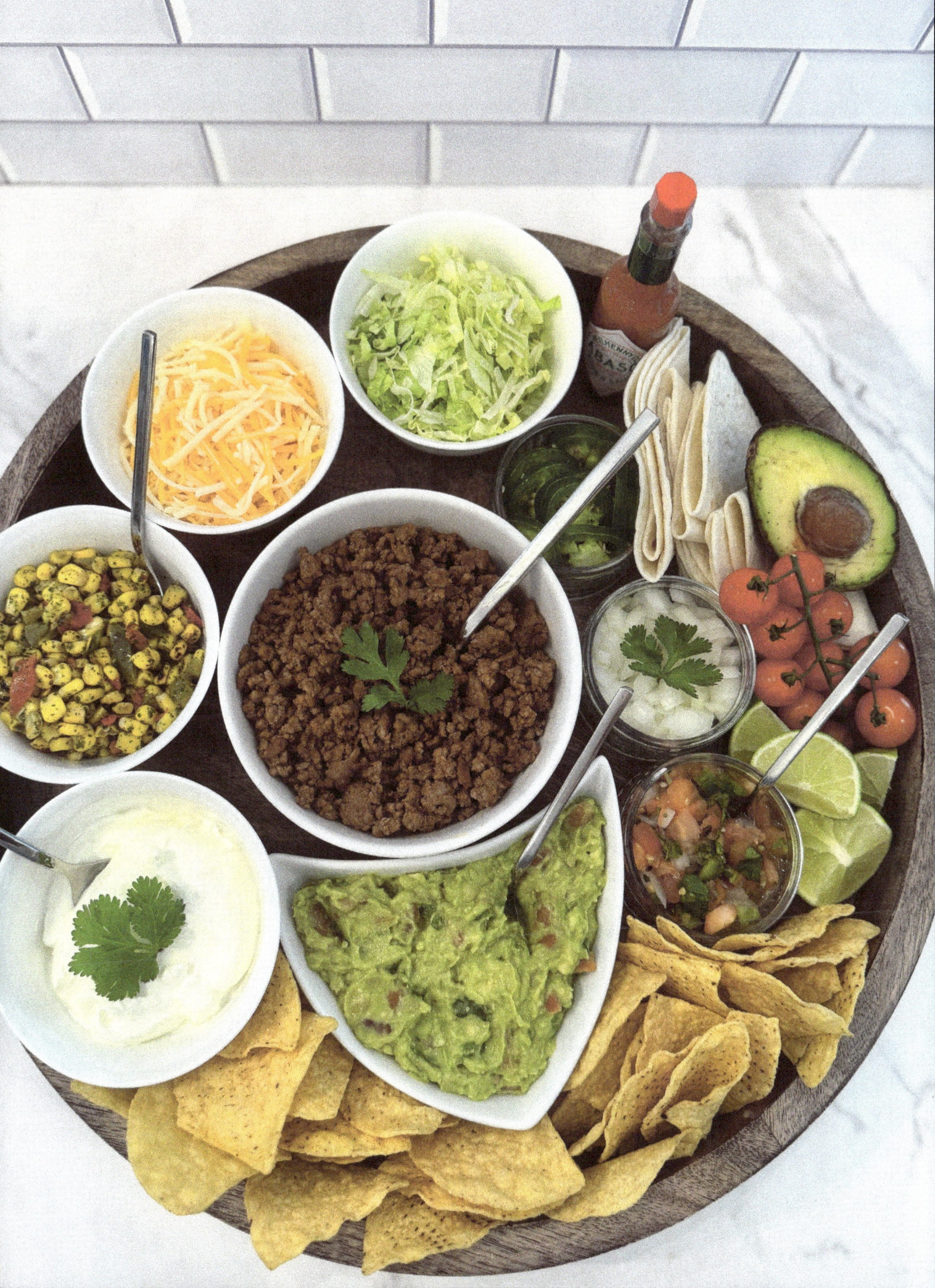

Burger Board

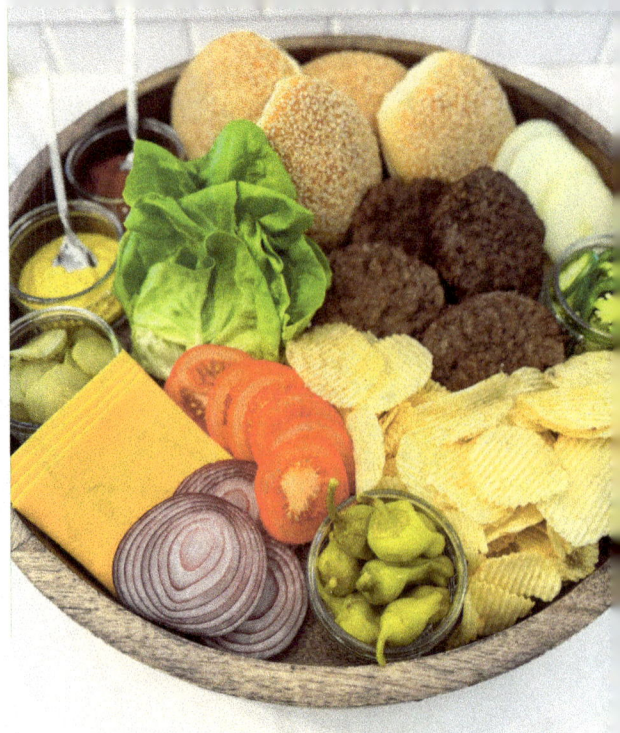

🌸 Preparation time
20 minutes

🍽 Serving
4

Ingredients:

- » 4 hamburger buns
- » 4 grilled hamburger patties
- » 4 slices cheddar cheese
- » 1/3 cup ketchup
- » 1/3 cup mustard
- » 1/3 cup mayonnaise (optional)
- » 4 lettuce leaves
- » 2 tomatoes, sliced
- » 1 red or white onion, sliced into rings
- » ½ cup sandwich pickles
- » ½ cup pepperoncini peppers
- » ½ cup sliced jalapeno
- » 1 cup potato chips

Instructions:

1. Grill the hamburger patties until cooked to your desired doneness.
2. Slice the tomatoes and onion into rings.
3. Prepare the lettuce leaves, sandwich pickles, pepperoncini peppers, and sliced jalapenos.
4. On a large board or platter, place the grilled hamburger patties in the center.
5. Arrange the hamburger buns around the patties.
6. Place the cheddar cheese slices next to the patties for easy access.
7. In small bowls or sections, arrange the ketchup, mustard, and mayo.
8. Arrange the lettuce leaves, tomato slices, and onion rings around the board.
9. Add the sandwich pickles, pepperoncini peppers, and sliced jalapenos.
10. Place the potato chips around the edges of the board.

Tips

1. Provide a variety of condiments like ketchup, mustard, and mayo for customization. This lets guests tailor their burgers to their liking.
2. Arrange ingredients like lettuce, tomato, and onion in separate rows for easy access. This keeps the board organized and visually appealing.

Nutrition facts (per serving)

| Calories: 950cal, | Carbs: 70g, | Protein: 35g, | Fat: 55g |

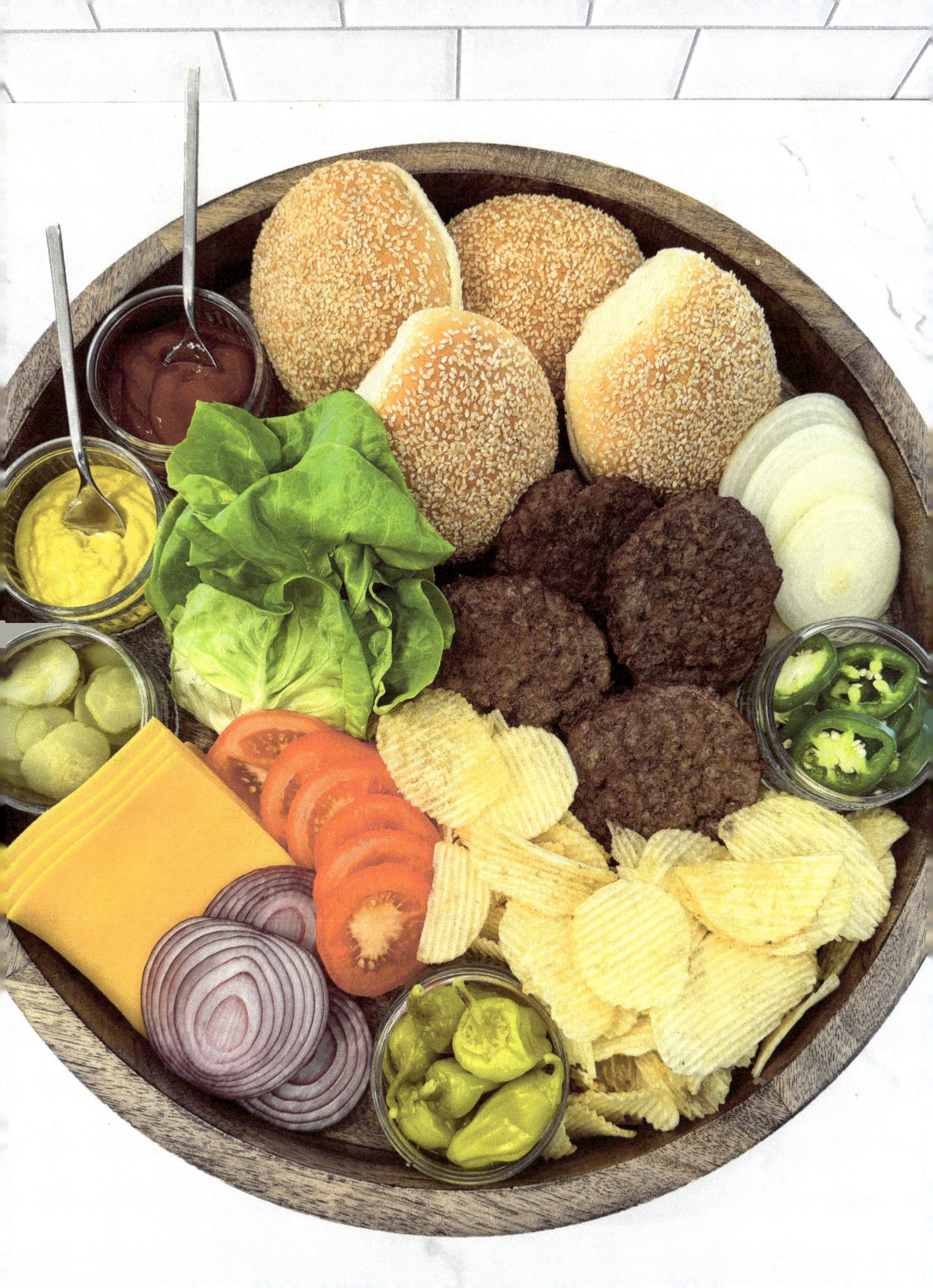

Submarine Sandwich Board

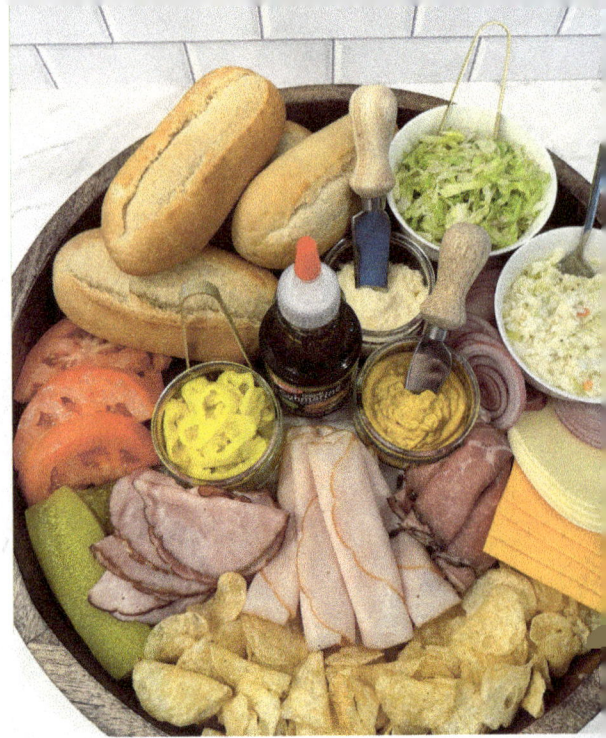

⚗ *Preparation time*
15 minutes

🍽 *Serving*
6

Ingredients:

» 4 baguette rolls, halved
» 2 sliced tomatoes
» 1 cup sliced pickles
» 1/2 lb sliced ham
» 1/2 lb sliced turkey
» 1/2 lb sliced roast beef
» 1/2 lb sliced cheddar cheese
» 1/2 lb sliced provolone cheese
» 1 cup shredded lettuce
» 1 cup coleslaw
» 1 cup sliced red onions
» 1 cup banana pepper rings
» 1/2 cup mayonnaise
» 1/2 cup mustard
» 4 cups potato chips

Instructions:

1. Halve the baguette rolls. Slice the tomatoes, pickles, and red onions.
2. Arrange the ham, turkey, roast beef, cheddar cheese, and provolone cheese in separate sections.
3. On a large board or platter, place the halved baguette rolls in the center.
4. Arrange the sliced tomatoes, pickles on the board. Place shredded lettuce, and coleslaw in the bowl.
5. Place the sliced red onions and banana pepper rings in separate sections.
6. Arrange the sliced ham, turkey, roast beef, cheddar cheese, and provolone cheese around the board. In small bowls, place the mayonnaise and mustard.
7. Add the potato chips around the edges of the board.
8. Serve immediately with small plates for easy sandwich assembly.

Tips
Include a selection of meats and cheeses to cater to different tastes. Arrange them neatly for easy sandwich assembly.

Nutrition facts (per serving)

Calories: 900cal,   Carbs: 85g,   Protein: 40g,   Fat: 55g

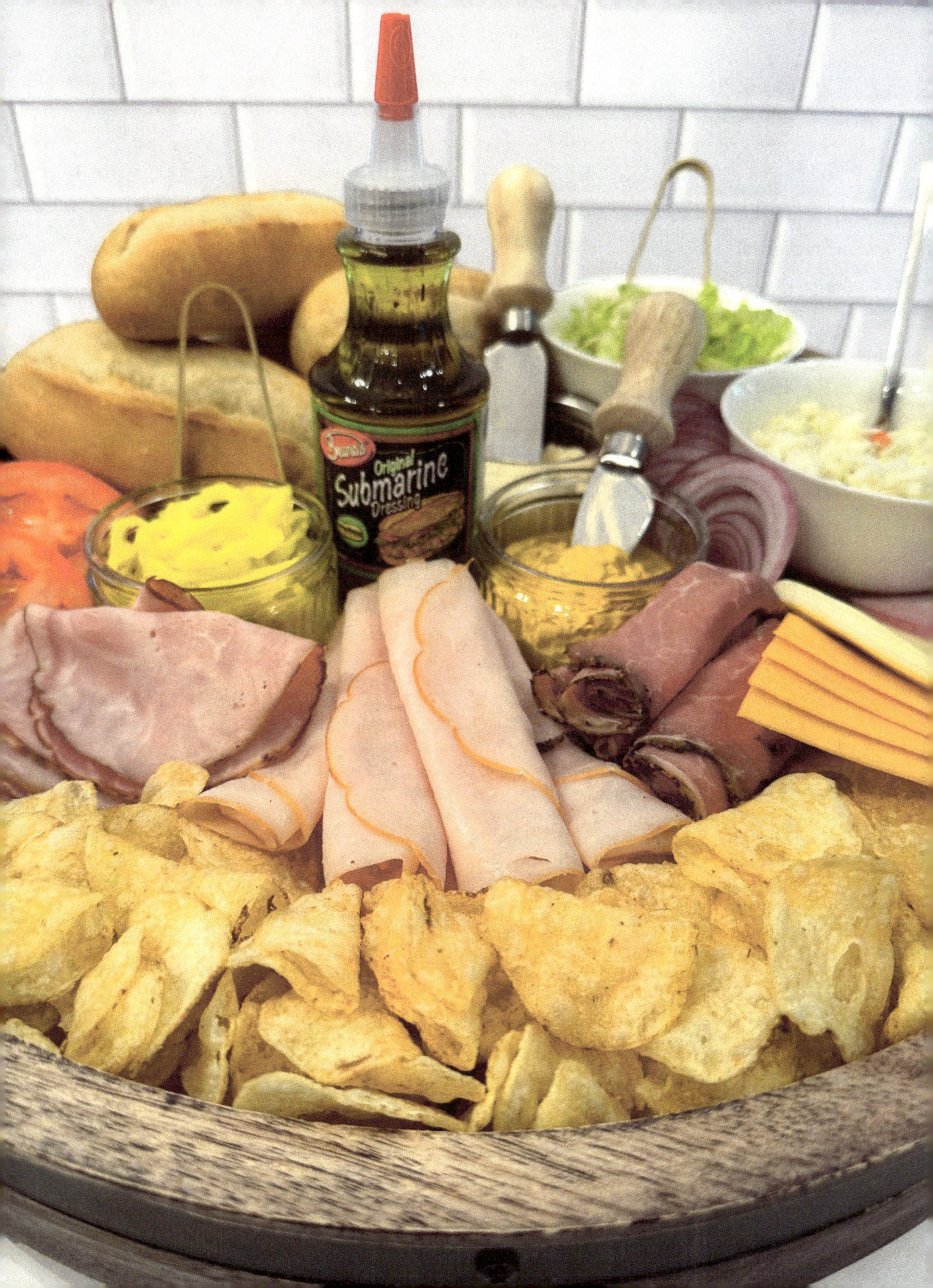

Mediterranean Board

%% Preparation time
30 minutes

🍽 Serving
8

Ingredients:

» 12 stuffed grape leaves (premade from the deli or canned)
» 1 lb grilled chicken kabobs or chunks
» 1 cup feta cheese chunks
» 1 cup chickpea hummus
» 1 cup roasted red pepper hummus
» 1 cup baba ghanouj
» 1/2 cup peppadew peppers
» 2 cups couscous or tabbouleh salad
» 1 cup black and green olive mix
» 1 cup sliced radishes
» 1 cup sliced cucumbers
» 1 cup cherry tomatoes
» 1 cup tzatziki sauce
» 1 lemon, cut into wedges
» 4 pita bread pockets, quartered or cut into triangles

Instructions:

1. Grill chicken kabobs or chunks until cooked through and slightly charred.
2. Quarter or cut pita bread pockets into triangles.
3. On a large board or platter, place the grilled chicken chunks or kabobs in the center.
4. Arrange the stuffed grape leaves around the chicken. Add the feta cheese chunks next to the grape leaves.
5. Arrange the baba ghanouj, roasted red pepper hummus, and chickpea hummus in little bowls around the platter.
6. Scatter the Peppadew peppers, black & green olive mix, radishes, cucumbers, and cherry tomatoes around the board.
7. Add the couscous or tabbouleh salad in a small bowl or section.
8. Place the tzatziki sauce in a bowl and add it to the board.
9. Arrange the lemon wedges and pita bread pockets around the edges of the board.
10. Serve immediately with small plates for easy dipping and assembling.

Tips Offer a variety of dips like hummus and baba ghanouj for a true Mediterranean experience. This allows guests to enjoy different flavors.

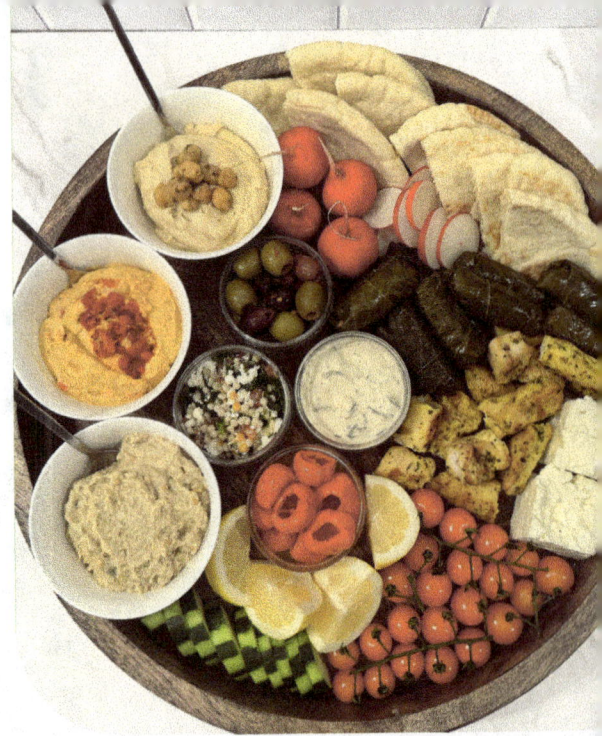

Nutrition facts (per serving)

Calories: 400cal,	Carbs: 35g,	Protein: 20g,	Fat: 21g

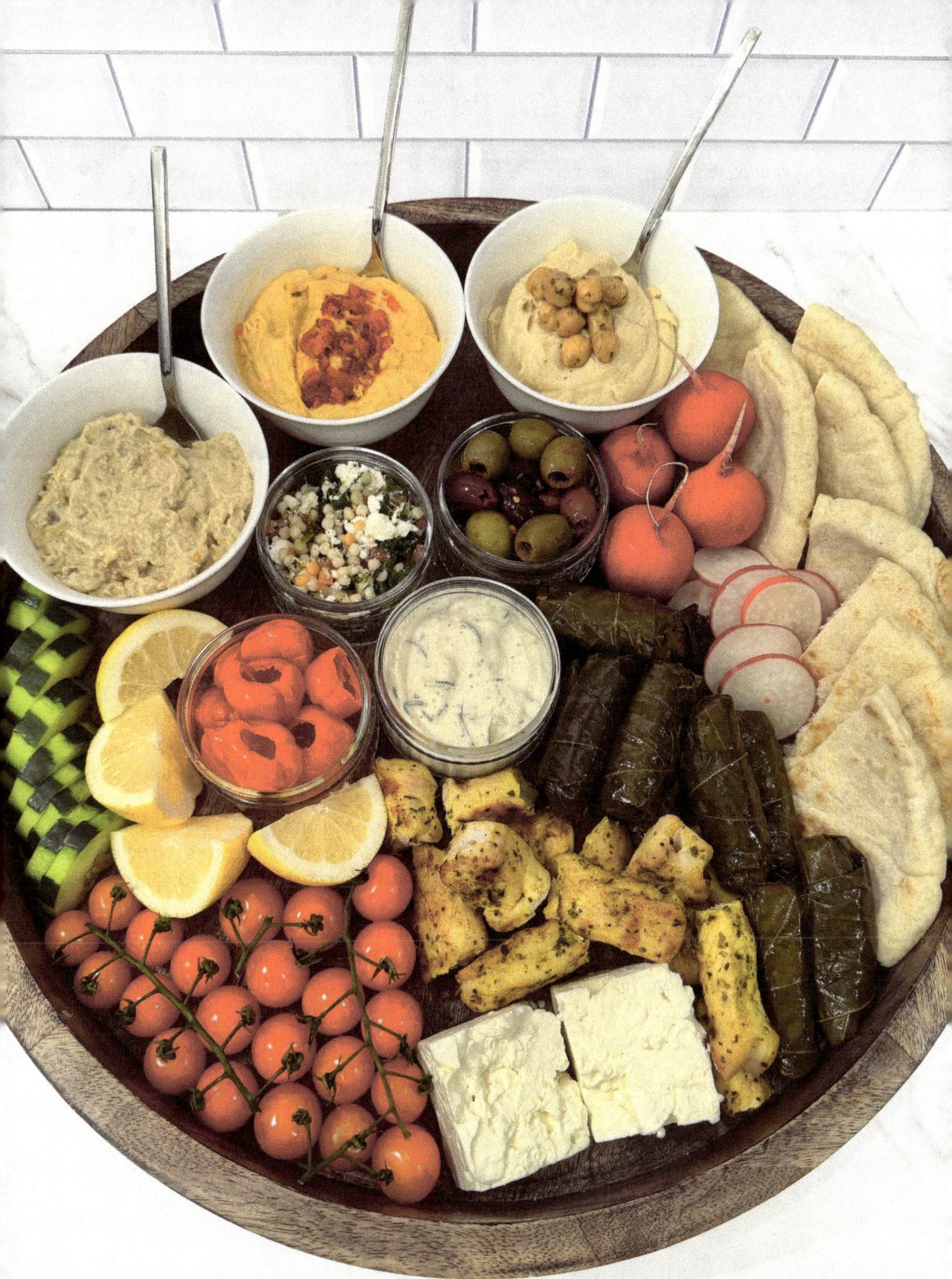

Chocolate Fondue Board

🎂 Preparation time 20 minutes

🍽 Serving 6

Ingredients:

» 10 madeleines
» 10 jumbo marshmallows
» 8 jumbo pretzels
» 6 strawberries, hulled
» 1/2 cup dried apricots
» 1/2 cup dried mango
» 6 rice krispie squares, cut into small pieces
» 1 1/2 cups melting or fondue chocolate
» 12 fondue sticks or food picks

Instructions:

1. Hull the strawberries and cut any large ones in half.
2. Cut the Rice Krispie squares into bite-sized pieces.
3. Arrange the madeleines, marshmallows, pretzels, dried apricots, dried mango, and Rice Krispie squares on a large platter or board.
4. Follow the directions on the fondue chocolate packaging to melt it. Usually, you may do this over a pot of simmering water in a heatproof bowl or fondue pot.
5. Transfer the melted chocolate to a fondue pot or heatproof bowl to keep warm.
6. Place the fondue pot or bowl in the center of the board.
7. Arrange the fondue sticks or food picks near the chocolate.
8. Make sure the dippers rice Krispie squares, marshmallows, pretzels, strawberries, dried apricots, and dried mango are conveniently located near the fondue pot.

Tips

To maintain the chocolate's melting consistency, use a small slow cooker or fondue pot. This guarantees a seamless and delightful dipping experience.

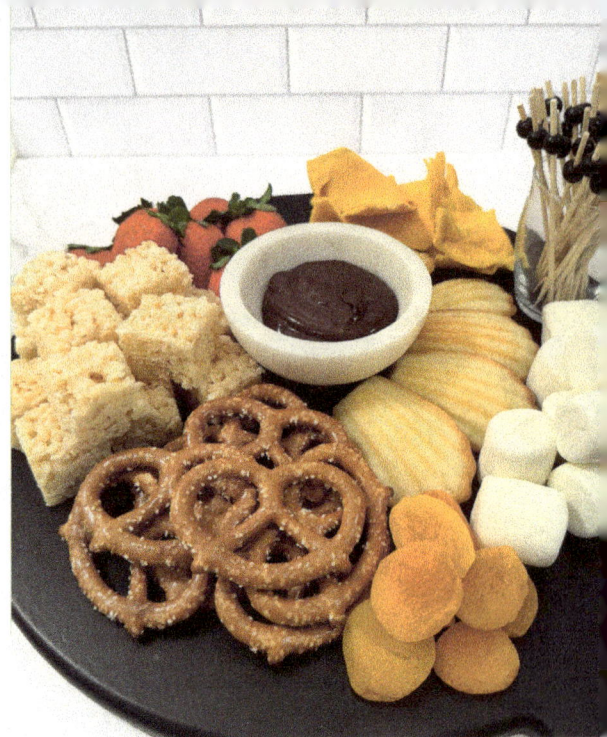

Nutrition facts (per serving)

Calories: 350cal,   Carbs: 50g,   Protein: 4g,   Fat: 15g

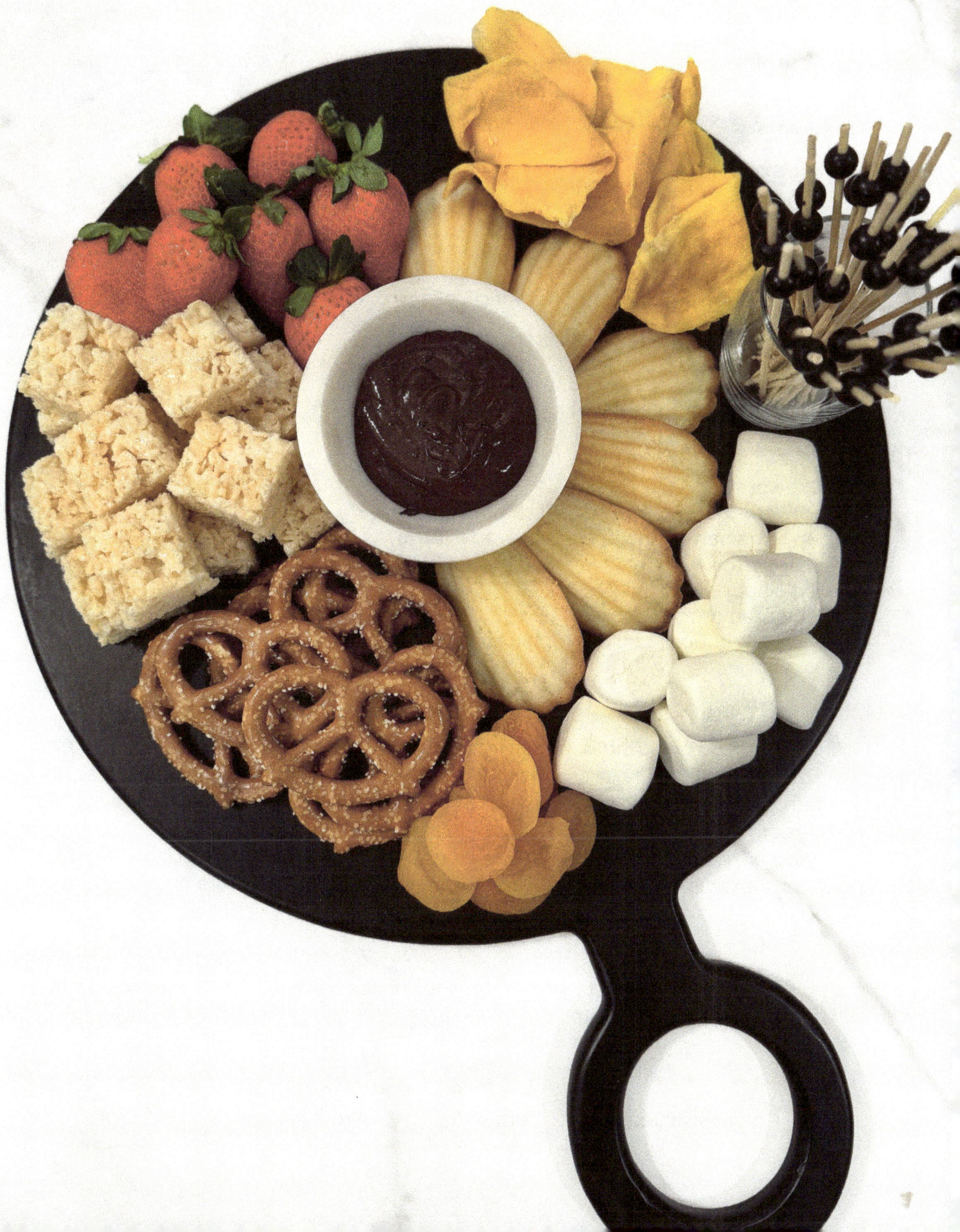

Skewer Board

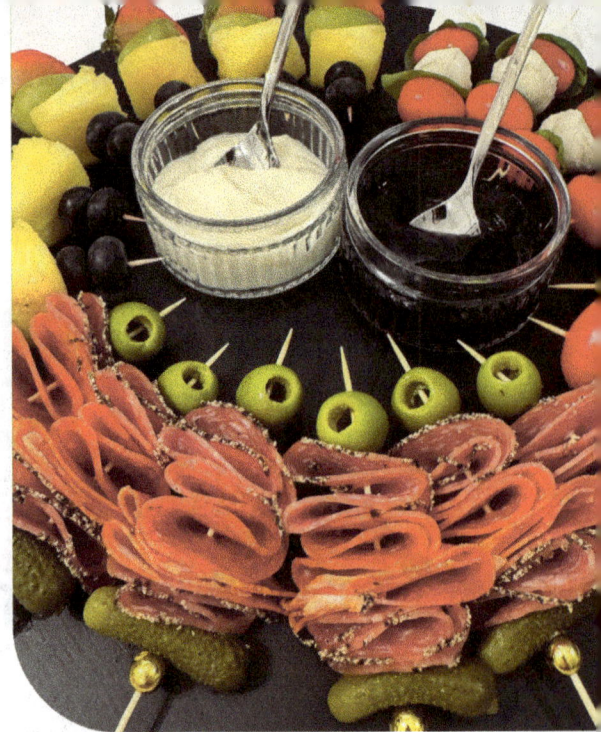

🍴 Preparation time
30 minutes

🍽 Serving
8

Ingredients:

Caprese Skewers
» 6 skewers
» 12 mozzarella balls (about 8 oz)
» 12 cherry tomatoes
» 6 fresh basil leaves
» 2 tbsp balsamic glaze (optional, for drizzling)

Salami Skewers
» 6 skewers
» 24 salami slices (about 4 oz)
» 6 olives or pickles (optional, for garnish)

Fruit Skewers
» 6 skewers
» 1 cup strawberries (hulled and halved if large)
» 12 blueberries
» 1 cup pineapple chunks
» 1 cup green grapes
» 4oz cream cheese fruit dip (optional, for dipping)

Instructions:

1. Thread 2 mozzarella balls, 2 cherry tomatoes, and 1 basil leaf onto each skewer. Drizzle with balsamic glaze if desired.
2. Alternate threading 2 salami slices and 2 cheese cubes onto each skewer. Add olives or pickles if desired.
3. Thread a mix of strawberries, melon, pineapple, and grapes onto each skewer.
4. Arrange the Caprese skewers, salami skewers, and fruit skewers on a large round board.

Tips Cut ingredients to similar sizes for uniform skewers. This ensures an even and balanced bite.

Nutrition facts (per serving)
Calories: 300cal,   Carbs: 17g,   Protein: 12g,   Fat: 13g

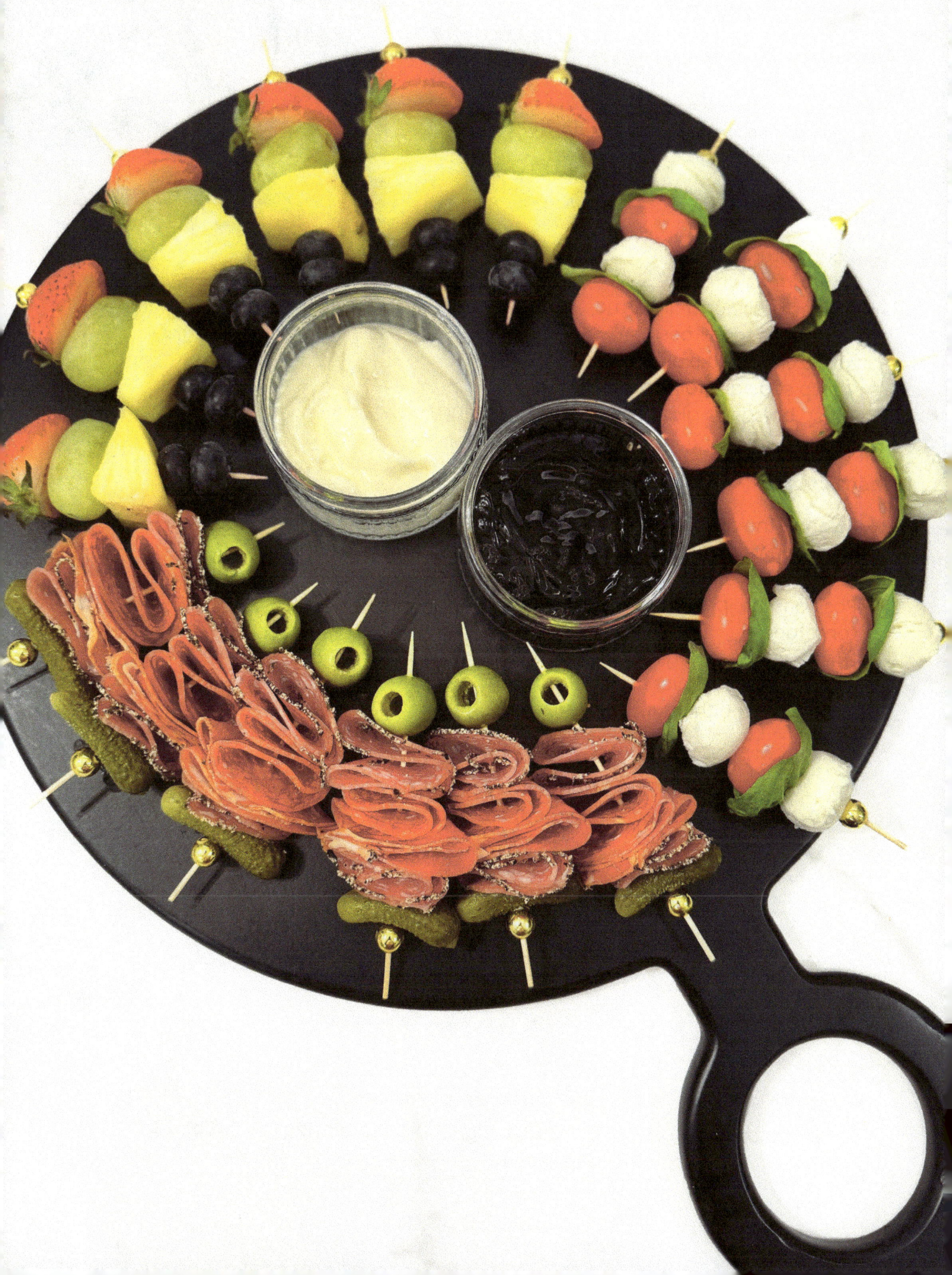

Burrata Heirloom Tomato Board

🕸 Preparation time
15 minutes

🍲 Serving
6

Ingredients:

» 4 cups arugula
» 8 oz burrata cheese
» 6 slices prosciutto di parma
» 4 heirloom tomatoes
» 2 tbsp extra virgin olive oil (for drizzling)
» 1/2 tsp sea salt (for sprinkling)
» 2 tbsp balsamic glaze (optional, for drizzling)

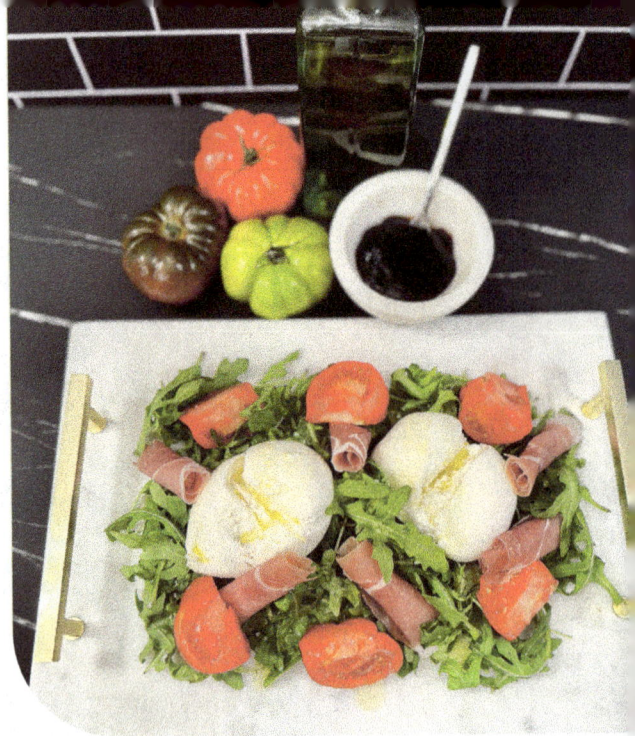

Instructions:

1. Arrange the arugula evenly on a large serving platter or board to create a bed.
2. Place the burrata cheese in the center of the arugula.
3. Drape the prosciutto slices around the burrata.
4. Position the prosciutto and burrata around the slices or wedges of heirloom tomatoes.
5. Drizzle the extra virgin olive oil evenly over the entire board.
6. Sprinkle sea salt over the burrata, tomatoes, and arugula.
7. If using, drizzle the balsamic glaze over the tomatoes and burrata.

Tips
Use ripe heirloom tomatoes for the best flavor. Their vibrant colors also enhance the visual appeal of the board.

Nutrition facts (per serving)

Calories: 210cal,   Carbs: 10g,   Protein: 12g,   Fat: 20g

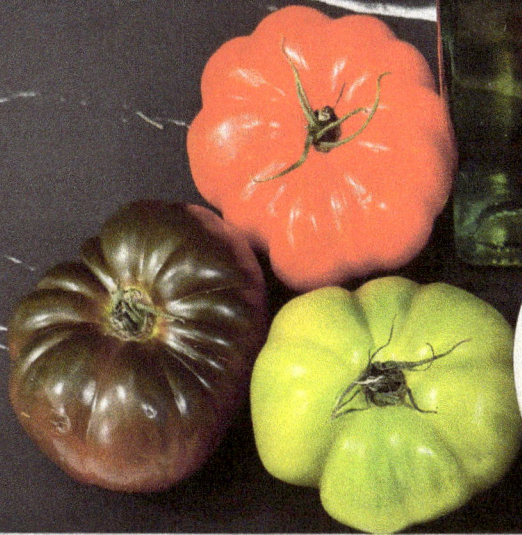

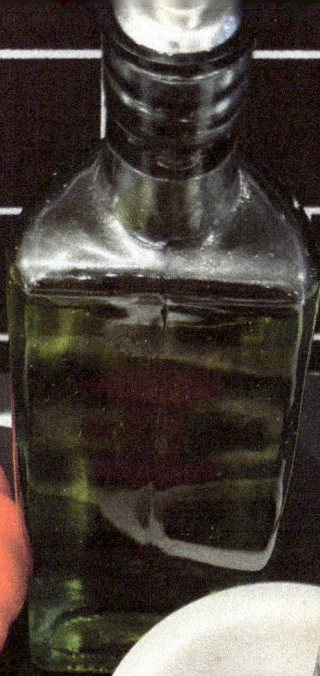

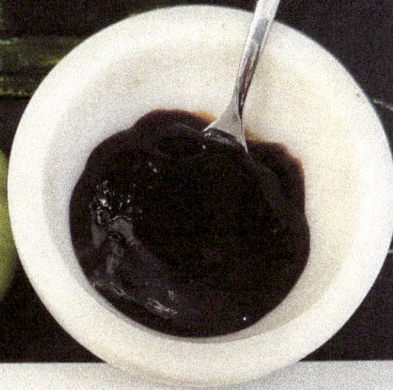

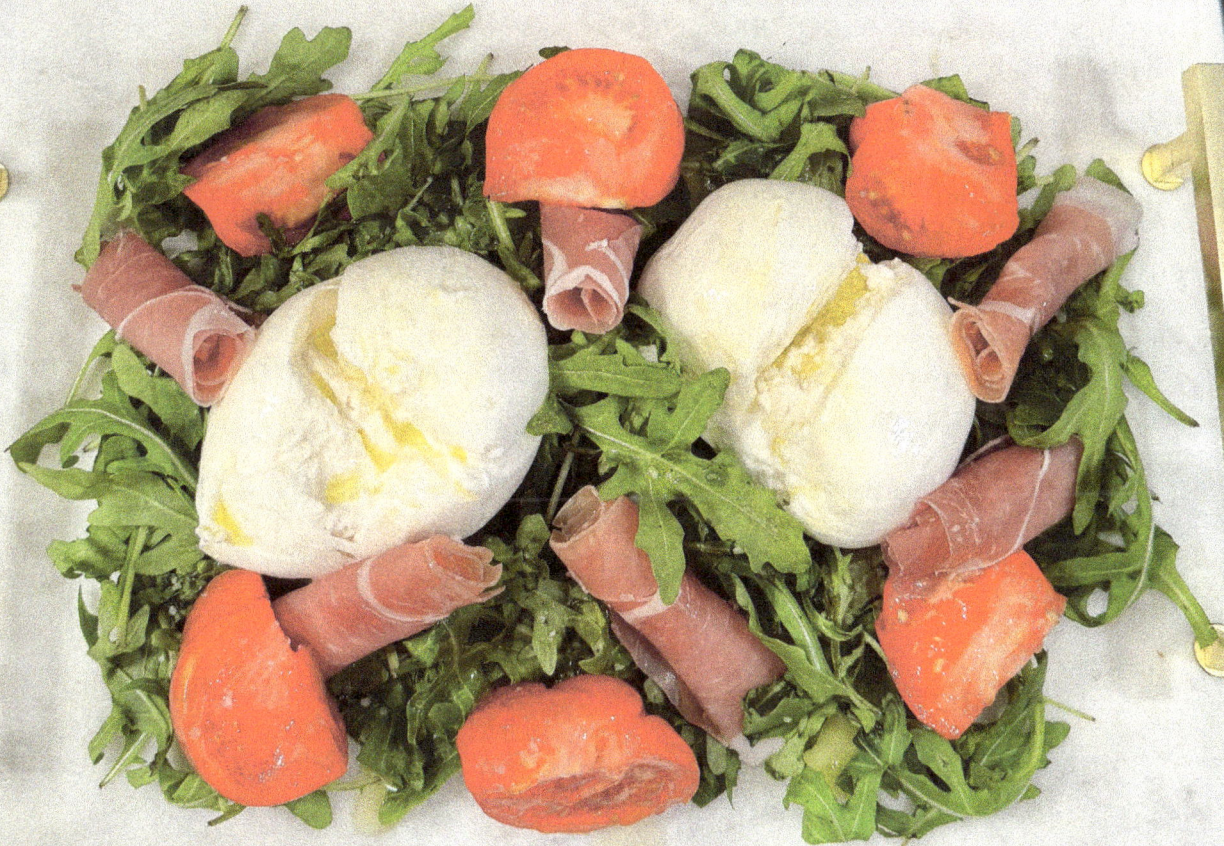

Sushi Hand Roll Board

🌸 Preparation time
15 minutes

🍽 Serving
6

Ingredients:

» 1 cup tuna poke
» 1 cup salmon poke
» 1 cup alaskan crab salad
» 2 cups sushi rice (cooked and seasoned)
» 10 sheets seaweed wrap
» 1 cup seaweed salad
» 1/2 cup wasabi peas
» 1/2 cup crispy onions
» 1 sliced avocado
» 1 sliced cucumber
» 1 cup masago (fish roe)
» 1/4 cup soy sauce
» 1/4 cup pickled ginger
» 1/4 cup spicy mayo
» 1/2 cup Nori seasoning (optional)
» 1/4 cup wasabi paste (optional)
» 1/2 cup Pocky sticks

Instructions:

1. Arrange the sushi rice in a bowl or on a small platter for easy access.
2. Place the tuna poke, salmon poke, and Alaskan crab salad in separate bowls or small dishes. Arrange the seaweed wraps on a large platter or board, cut in half to make hand rolls.
3. Slice the avocado and cucumber and place them on the board.
4. Arrange the seaweed salad, wasabi peas, crispy onions, and masago in small bowls.
5. Place the soy sauce, pickled ginger, spicy mayo, and wasabi paste in small dishes for dipping.
6. Add the Nori seasoning and Pocky sticks for garnish and a sweet touch.
7. Arrange all items on a large board or platter in an organized manner for easy access.
8. Make sure to place the dipping sauces and optional items where they are easily reachable.

Tips

Use the freshest fish possible for poke and sushi. In addition to encouraging diners to assemble their own hand rolls to preserve the freshness of the ingredients, this guarantees the greatest flavor and texture. Offer a selection of toppings and fillings to allow for personalization.

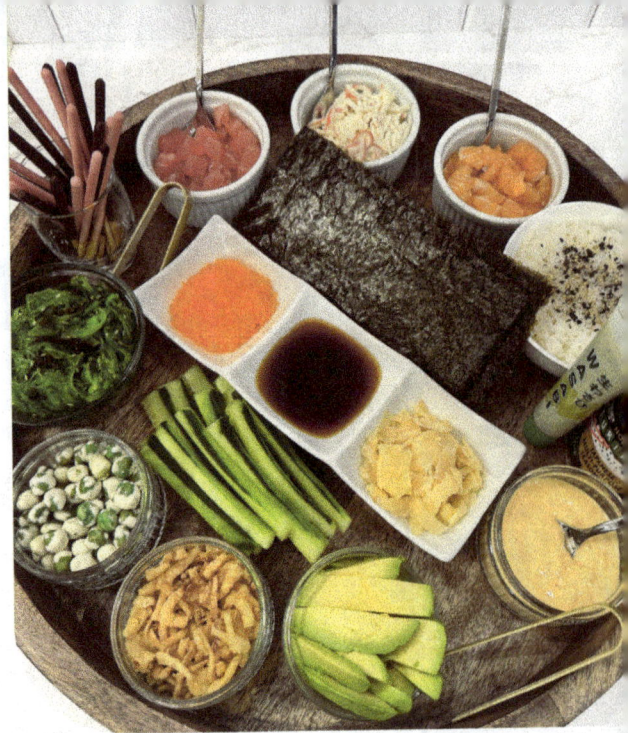

Nutrition facts (per serving)

Calories: 350cal,	Carbs: 35g,	Protein: 15g,	Fat: 15g

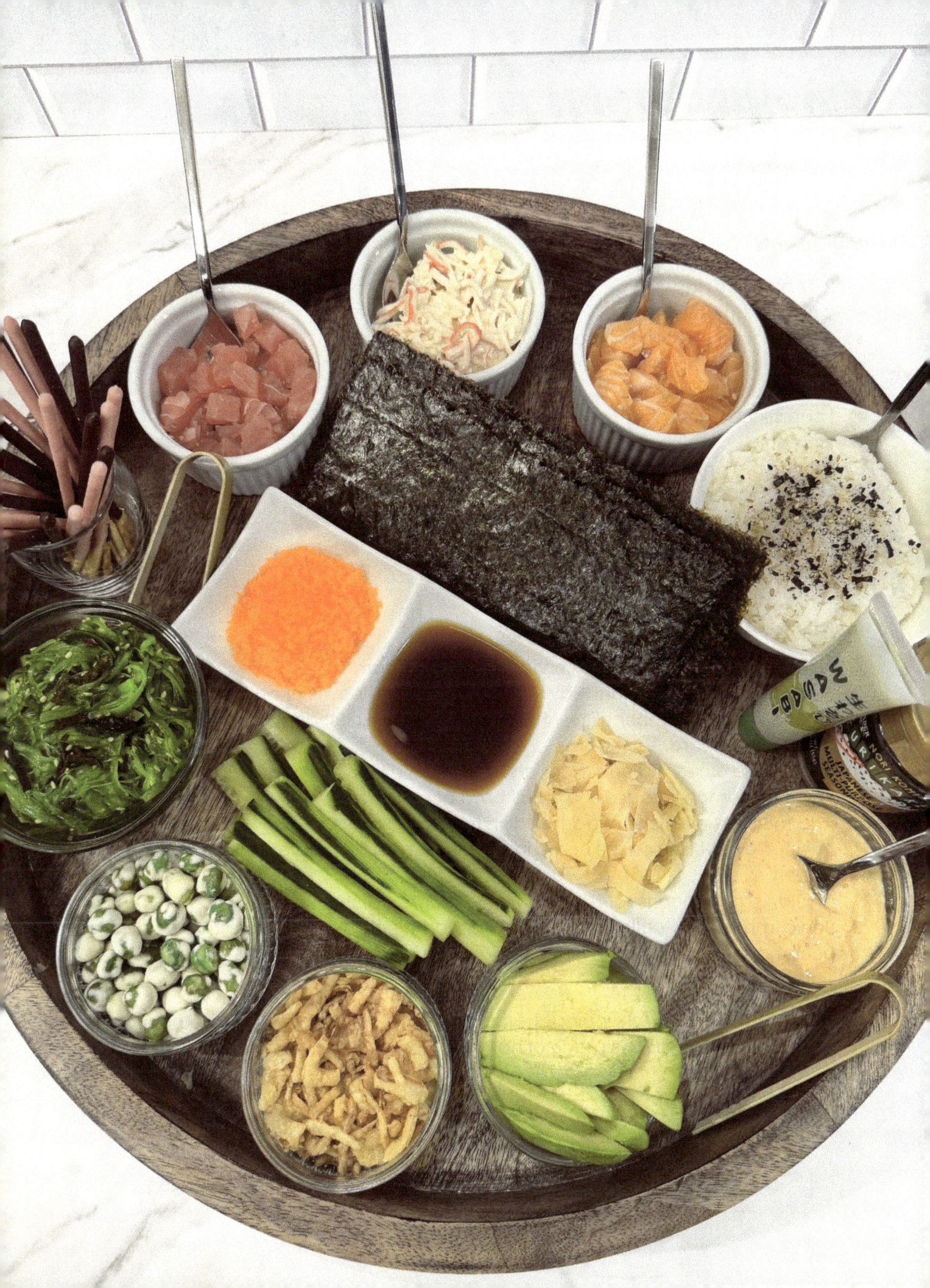

Caviar Board

% Preparation time
   20 minutes

🍽 Serving
   6

Ingredients:

» 2 oz black caviar
» 2 oz salmon caviar
» 6 oz smoked salmon (sliced)
» 4 hard-boiled eggs (sliced)
» 12 blini (small pancakes)
» 1 cup sliced cucumber
» 1 lemon
» 1/2 cup red onion (diced)
» 1/4 cup capers
» 1/2 cup crème fraîche
» 1/4 cup fresh dill (chopped)
» 1/4 cup chives (chopped)

Instructions:

1. Arrange the blini on a large serving platter or board.
2. Place the black caviar and salmon caviar in small bowls or on the board.
3. Arrange the cucumber slices, hard-boiled egg slices, and smoked salmon slices around the board.
4. Scatter the diced red onion, capers, and fresh dill on the board.
5. Place the lemon wedges in a small bowl or on the board.
6. Add the crème fraîche in a small dish for easy access.
7. Arrange everything on the board in a neat manner, leaving room for guests to select what they want.
8. Provide small spoons for the caviar and crème fraîche.
9. Serve immediately, allowing guests to assemble their own bites with the caviar and accompaniments.

Tips
To prevent changing the flavor of the caviar, serve it with non-metallic cutlery. Spoons made of horn, bone, or mother-of-pearl work well.

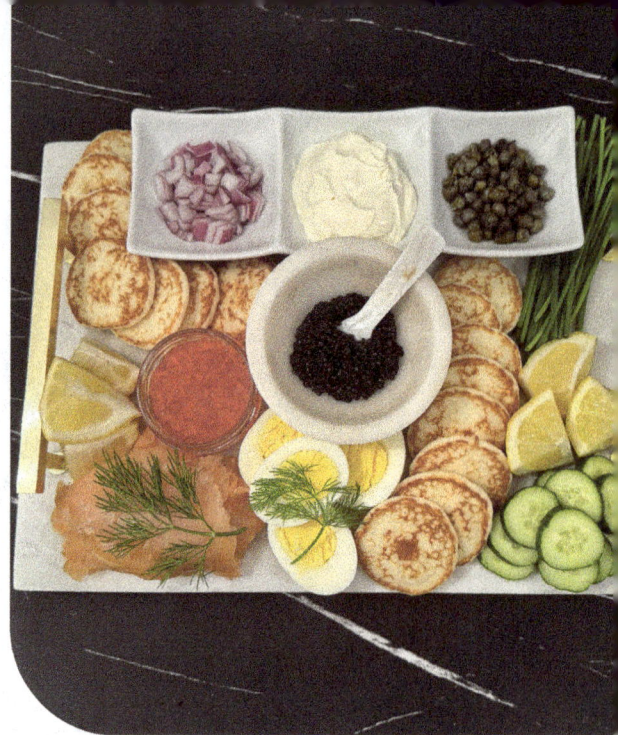

Nutrition facts (per serving)

Calories: 250cal,   Carbs: 12g,   Protein: 16g,   Fat: 15g

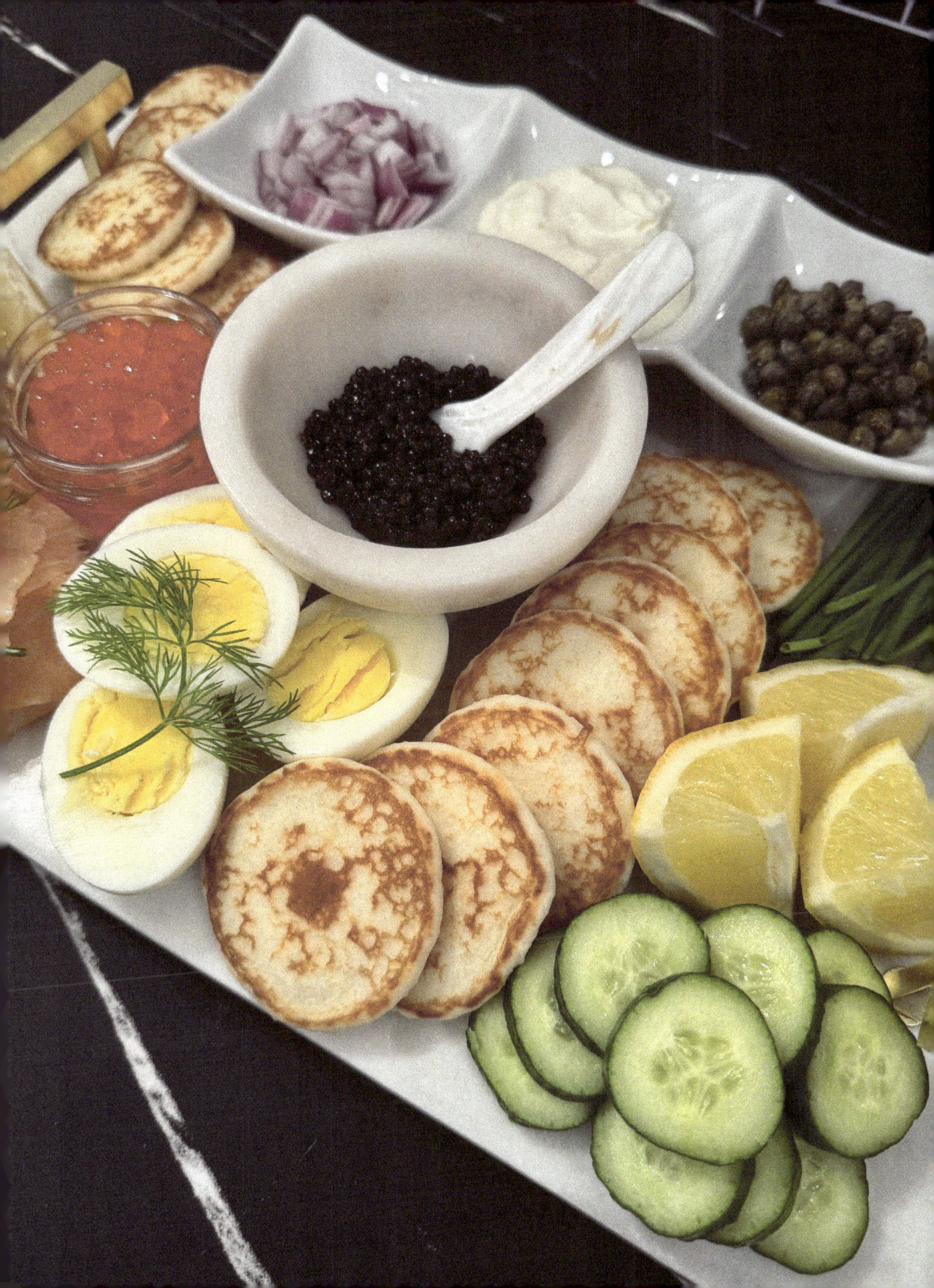

General Tips

1 Make sure the flavours and textures are balanced; there should be equal amounts of crunchy, creamy, salty, sweet, and fresh ingredients.

2 Visual appeal is key. Arrange items attractively and use garnishes like herbs or flowers to enhance the look.

3 Estimate about 2-3 oz of meat or cheese per person for charcuterie and cheese boards. For other boards, portion according to the expected serving size and appetite of your guests.

4 When feasible, pre-cut the ingredients to facilitate guests' selection. Additionally, this saves time on the day of the event.

5 Use the freshest ingredients possible. This is especially important for fruits, vegetables, and seafood.

6 Incorporate seasonal produce for the best flavors and variety. It's also a great way to keep your boards exciting throughout the year.

7 Think about labelling any cheeses, meats, or dips you're serving so your visitors know what to choose.

8 Provide appropriate utensils like cheese knives, small spoons, tongs, and forks to make serving easier.

9 Use garnishes not only for flavor but also to fill gaps on the board and create a fuller look. Fresh herbs, nuts, and edible flowers are excellent choices.

10 To bring out the flavours of meats and cheeses, serve them room temperature. Before serving, remove them from the refrigerator 30 to 45 minutes in advance.

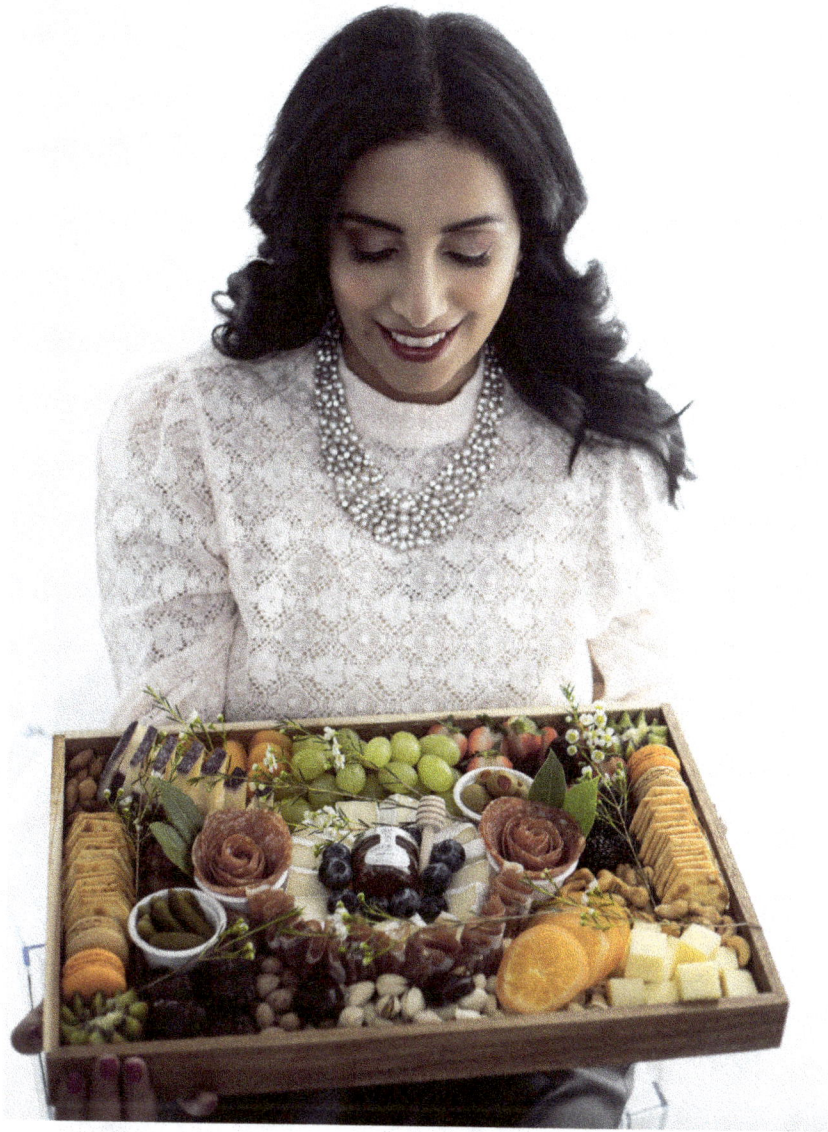

Thank you

www.ingramcontent.com/pod-product-compliance
Lightning Source LLC
Chambersburg PA
CBHW080428030426
42335CB00020B/2631